Lecture Notes in Computer Science **16474**

The series Lecture Notes in Computer Science (LNCS), including its subseries Lecture Notes in Artificial Intelligence (LNAI) and Lecture Notes in Bioinformatics (LNBI), has established itself as a medium for the publication of new developments in computer science and information technology research, teaching, and education.

LNCS enjoys close cooperation with the computer science R & D community, the series counts many renowned academics among its volume editors and paper authors, and collaborates with prestigious societies. Its mission is to serve this international community by providing an invaluable service, mainly focused on the publication of conference and workshop proceedings and postproceedings. LNCS commenced publication in 1973.

Juan P. Wachs · Andrew W. Kirkpatrick ·
Guillaume Landry · Tom Julius Bloecker
Editors

AI for Real-Time Tumor Tracking in MRI-Guided Radiotherapy and Trauma Procedure Understanding

TrackRAD2025 Challenge
and Second Trauma Thompson Challenge
Held in Conjunction with MICCAI 2025
Daejeon, South Korea, September 23 and 27, 2025
Proceedings

Springer

Editors
Juan P. Wachs
Purdue University
West Lafayette, IN, USA

Andrew W. Kirkpatrick
Alberta Health Services
Calgary, AB, Canada

Guillaume Landry
LMU University Hospital
Munich, Germany

Tom Julius Bloecker
LMU University Hospital
Munich, Germany

ISSN 0302-9743 ISSN 1611-3349 (electronic)
Lecture Notes in Computer Science
ISBN 978-3-032-35045-9 ISBN 978-3-032-35046-6 (eBook)
https://doi.org/10.1007/978-3-032-35046-6

This Springer imprint is published by the registered company Springer Nature Switzerland AG
The registered company address is: Gewerbestrasse 11, 6330 Cham, Switzerland

TrackRAD2025 Preface

Magnetic resonance imaging (MRI)-guided radiotherapy (MRIgRT) integrates MRI with linear accelerators (MRI-linacs), enabling real-time motion management based on temporally resolved 2D MRI (cine-MRI). For this purpose, radiotherapy targets (typically the gross tumor volume) need to be located in these frames, in real time, to support precise and efficient delivery methods.

The TrackRAD2025 challenge was organized to provide the first public, multi-institutional dataset and evaluation platform to benchmark algorithms for MRIgRT target tracking in 2D+t cine-MRI. Participants had to create algorithms that generate a tumor segmentation mask for every frame in a sequence, starting from a given ground truth segmentation mask in the first frame. The dataset comprised sagittal cine-MRI scans of 585 cancer patients undergoing radiotherapy with 0.35 T and 1.5 T MRI-linacs at six different institutions, providing more than 2,878,000 unlabeled cine-MRI frames and expert-annotated targets in more than 10,000 labeled frames from 108 sequences. The target sites included the thorax, abdomen, and pelvis. The algorithms submitted by the participants were executed on the challenge platform and assessed using metrics in three categories: geometric accuracy, surrogate dose accuracy, and execution speed. The ranking was derived using a Rank-Then-Mean scheme.

In total, TrackRAD2025 attracted 148 registrations from 28 countries, 100 preliminary submissions, and 24 final submissions from 14 teams. The submissions highlight the interest in MRIgRT and artificial intelligence solutions for the associated tasks. The top five methods achieved mean Dice similarity coefficients >0.87 and Euclidean center distances <2.1 mm, comparable to interobserver variability. These solutions featured promptable foundation models, four fine-tuned Segment Anything Model 2 (SAM2) variants, and one used CoTracker off the shelf, highlighting the relevance of these models for medical imaging tasks.

In addition to enabling this benchmarking and evaluation, TrackRAD2025 also supported the application of MRIgRT target tracking and motion management more broadly. To encourage engagement, the challenge was promoted at ESTRO 2025 on May 4, 2025. The challenge concluded with a workshop at the 28th International Conference on Medical Image Computing and Computer Assisted Intervention (MICCAI 2025) on September 23, 2025. These venues provided an opportunity to bridge the computer science and medical physics communities. In a similar spirit, the participants were offered the opportunity to have their reports published as a joint LNCS volume alongside the Trauma THOMPSON challenge 2025 on real-time AI-assisted remote instruction systems, highlighting a different time-critical task within the medical field. Seven submissions were received for this volume, and all were accepted after a single-blind review process in which they received two reviews each, on average.

For more information on the challenge and its results, visit the official TrackRAD2025 website at https://trackrad2025.grand-challenge.org.

April 2026

Guillaume Landry
Tom Julius Bloecker

The Trauma THOMPSON Challenge 2025 Preface

The landscape of artificial intelligence has continued to evolve toward the provision of proactive assistance in high-stakes human activities. From autonomous robots to complex surgical interventions, the role of AI agents as mentors and assistants is becoming increasingly central to modern technological progress. Building on the success of the inaugural challenge held in 2023, the Trauma THOMPSON Challenge 2025 represented a significant advancement in the application of computer vision and machine learning to the critical domains of field and humanitarian medicine. While many activity recognition benchmarks focus on everyday scenarios like cooking or sports, this challenge remains uniquely positioned to address the acute technical requirements of recognizing and predicting life-saving interventions in uncontrolled, field-based, and austere environments.

The primary objective of the 2025 iteration remained the development of robust algorithms capable of real-time activity understanding during medical emergencies. Such capabilities are essential for creating intelligent medical mentors or assistants that can support inexperienced paramedics and combat medics long before a patient reaches a definitive care facility. The dataset leveraged high-resolution egocentric video recordings of essential lifesaving procedures, including cricothyroidotomy, tube thoracostomy, needle thoracostomy, intraosseous infusion, and tourniquet application. By representing medical actions through verb-noun pairs and temporal segmentations, the challenge pushed the boundaries of open-set classification and action anticipation with unseen actions in the test sets, forcing participants to develop models that generalize across diverse environments and understand medical actions instead of memorizing scenes.

Reflecting the growing importance of this research area, the 2025 challenge attracted a cohort of 75 total participants. The first task within the development phase received 29 submissions, while the second task drew 22 submissions, and the fourth task recorded 3 submissions. This momentum carried forward into the final test phase, where the community demonstrated its rigor and commitment to benchmarking performance. The final test phase for the second task maintained a strong participation level with 22 submissions, while the first and fourth tasks concluded with 7 and 3 submissions respectively. This high level of activity underscores the commitment of the global research community to refining AI models for the complexities of prehospital care.

The results and technical insights generated during this event were showcased at the 28th International Conference on Medical Image Computing and Computer Assisted Intervention (MICCAI 2025). This venue provided a vital platform for interdisciplinary dialogue between computer vision specialists and medical professionals, ensuring that the proposed algorithmic solutions remain firmly grounded in clinical utility. Furthermore, the challenge papers are published as a joint LNCS volume alongside the MICCAI 2025 TrackRAD2025 challenge on Real-Time Tumor Tracking for MRI-guided Radiotherapy, which highlights complementary machine learning perspectives within the medical field. Five submissions were received for this volume, and all five were accepted after a single-blind review procedure in which they received three reviews each, on average. The organizers wish to express their profound gratitude to the participants, the reviewers, and the broader MICCAI community for their dedication to improving survival outcomes through the fusion of medicine and artificial intelligence. For more information regarding the challenge and its outcomes, please visit our official Trauma THOMPSON Challenge 2025 website at https://t3challenge25.grand-challenge.org.

April 2026

Yupeng Zhuo
Andrew W. Kirkpatrick
Juan P. Wachs

Organization

General Chair of TrackRAD2025

Guillaume Landry	LMU University Hospital, Munich, Germany

Program Committee of TrackRAD2025

Adrian Thummerer	LMU University Hospital, Munich, Germany
Christopher Kurz	LMU University Hospital, Munich, Germany
Coen Hurkmans	Catharina Hospital, The Netherlands
Davide Cusumano	Mater Olbia Hospital, Italy
Denis Dudáš	LMU University Hospital, Munich, Germany
Elia Lombardo	LMU University Hospital, Munich, Germany
Guillaume Landry	LMU University Hospital, Munich, Germany
Hilary Byrne	GenesisCare Sydney, Australia
Lorenzo Placidi	Policlinic Gemelli, Italy
Marco Fusella	Policlinico Abano, Italy
Marco Riboldi	LMU Munich, Germany
Matteo Maspero	UMC Utrecht, The Netherlands
Michael Jameson	GenesisCare Sydney, Australia
Miguel Palacios	Amsterdam UMC, The Netherlands
Paul Keall	University of Sydney, Australia
Pim Borman	UMC Utrecht, The Netherlands
Rob Tijssen	Catharina Hospital, The Netherlands
Tom Blöcker	LMU University Hospital, Munich, Germany
Yiling Wang	Sichuan Cancer Hospital, China

Data Contributors of TrackRAD2025

Martijn Intven	UMC Utrecht, The Netherlands
Pim Borman	UMC Utrecht, The Netherlands
Yiling Wang	Sichuan Cancer Hospital, China
Yu Fan	Sichuan Cancer Hospital, China
Yue Zhao	Sichuan Cancer Hospital, China
Miguel Palacios	Amsterdam UMC, The Netherlands
Paul Cobussen	Amsterdam UMC, The Netherlands

Tobias Finazzi	Amsterdam UMC, The Netherlands
Shyama U. Tetar	Amsterdam UMC, The Netherlands
Cornelis J.A. Haasbeek	Amsterdam UMC, The Netherlands
Elia Lombardo	LMU University Hospital, Munich, Germany
Guillaume Landry	LMU University Hospital, Munich, Germany
Christopher Kurz	LMU University Hospital, Munich, Germany
Christianna Iris Papadopoulou	LMU University Hospital, Munich, Germany
Rob Tijssens	Catharina Hospital, The Netherlands
Coen Hurkmans	Catharina Hospital, The Netherlands
Hilary Byrne	GenesisCare, Australia
Michael Jameson	GenesisCare, Australia

General Chair of the Trauma THOMPSON Challenge 2025

Yupeng Zhuo	Purdue University, USA

Program Committee Chairs of the Trauma THOMPSON Challenge 2025

Andrew W. Kirkpatrick	University of Calgary, Canada
Juan Wachs	Purdue University, IU School of Medicine, USA

Program Committee of the Trauma THOMPSON Challenge 2025

Eddie Zhang	Purdue University, USA
Xiangchen	Purdue University, USA
Aditya Pachpande	Purdue University, USA
Jessica McKee	University of Calgary, Canada
Edgar Rojas-Muñoz	Texas A&M University, USA
Brian VanVoorst	RTX BBN Technologies, USA
Jin Tae Kwak	Korea University, South Korea
Stas Tiomkin	Texas Tech University, USA
Vikhyat Bebarta	University of Colorado Anschutz Medical Campus, USA
Yanjun Gao	University of Colorado Anschutz Medical Campus, USA

Data Contributors of the Trauma THOMPSON Challenge 2025

Kyle Couperus	Geneva Foundation, Madigan Army Medical Center, USA
Christopher Colombo	Geneva Foundation, Madigan Army Medical Center, USA
Oanh Tran	Geneva Foundation, Madigan Army Medical Center, USA
Jonah Beck	Geneva Foundation, Madigan Army Medical Center, USA
DeAnna DeVane	Geneva Foundation, Madigan Army Medical Center, USA
Andrew W. Kirkpatrick	University of Calgary, Canada
Jessica McKee	University of Calgary, Canada
Ross Candelore	Madigan Army Medical Center, USA
Chad Gorbatkin	Madigan Army Medical Center, USA
Eleanor Birch	Madigan Army Medical Center, USA

Contents

TrackRAD 2025

The Trauma THOMPSON Challenge 2025

TrackRAD 2025

A Three-Stage Semi-supervised Fine-Tuning Method for SAM2 in Real-Time MRI Tumor Segmentation

Kailin He, Shengqian Zhu, Ying Song, Guangjun Li, and Junjie Hu(✉)

Machine Intelligence Laboratory College of Computer Science, Sichuan University, Chengdu 610065, China
hujunjie@scu.edu.cn

Abstract. In the TrackRAD2025 challenge, we propose a three-stage semi-supervised fine-tuning method for real-time MRI tumor segmentation based on Segment Anything Model 2 (SAM2). Our approach employs the `sam2_hiera_tiny` variant as the backbone network, which is applied uniformly across all anatomical locations and field strengths. The core of our methodology is a progressive learning strategy: (1) we first perform supervised full-parameter fine-tuning on 38 labeled cases; (2) the trained model is then used to generate high-quality pseudo-labels for 100 unlabeled cases; (3) finally, we conduct a second round of fine-tuning on the combined set of labeled and pseudo-labeled data to enhance generalization. For data preprocessing, `.mha` files were converted to JPGs, normalized with min–max scaling, and cropped to an input size of 512×512. Standard geometric and color augmentations are also applied. The model is optimized using AdamW with a cosine decay learning rate schedule, initialized at 2.0×10^{-7}. The loss function was a weighted combination of mask, Dice, class, and IoU losses. The final model submitted was selected based on its superior performance on a comprehensive set of metrics on a local validation set of 12 cases. On the official test set, our method achieved a DSC of 0.8860 (second place) and a relative D98 dose of 0.963 (first place), achieving second place in the challenge. The code is available at https://github.com/togetherhkl/TrackRAD2025.

Keywords: SAM2 · TrackRAD2025 · Tumor tracking · MRI-guided Radiotherapy

1 Introduction

Magnetic Resonance Imaging-guided Radiotherapy (MRIgRT) enables real-time monitoring of motion trajectories for tumors and organs at risk (OARs) through dynamic imaging. This capability provides the technical foundation for Adaptive Radiotherapy (ART) [1,2]. A major bottleneck in clinical translation is the

---

J. Hu and G. Li—are the co-corresponding authors.

J. P. Wachs et al. (Eds.): TrackRAD/TTC 2025, LNCS 16474, pp. 3–16, 2027.
https://doi.org/10.1007/978-3-032-35046-6_1

lack of automated algorithms that can rapidly and accurately segment tumor contours in continuous cine-MRI sequences. This limitation is exacerbated by three primary challenges: (1) **Motion Complexity**: Three-dimensional non-rigid deformations induced by physiological activity hinder conventional 2D real-time MRI from accurately modeling target motion. High-precision segmentation within milliseconds is required to meet the stringent real-time demands of ART [1]. (2) **Image Heterogeneity**: Variations in equipment types (e.g., 1.5T/0.35T), scanning parameters, and inter-patient differences result in fluctuating image contrast, which reduces the robustness of segmentation algorithms [3]. (3) **Scarcity of Labeled Data**: The high cost of expert delineation and the resulting small sample sizes limit the development of generalizable deep learning models [4,5].

The emergence of foundation models provides a novel framework to tackle this challenge. Foundation models are large-scale models generally pre-trained on extensive datasets using self-supervised learning, allowing adaptation to a wide range of downstream tasks [6]. Their adaptability and accuracy can be further improved by providing different types of input prompts or by fine-tuning on specific task data [7]. Compared to traditional large models, foundation models offer several advantages: pre-training costs are amortized across multiple downstream tasks, which reduces overall energy consumption [8]; they require only minimal labeled data for fine-tuning on specific tasks [9]; and their smaller number of parameters makes them more suitable for deployment on edge devices [10].

Segment Anything Model 2 (SAM2) is a next-generation promptable foundation model for real-time video segmentation that builds upon the strong image segmentation capabilities of its predecessor. By pre-training on large and diverse image and video datasets, SAM2 learns rich and generalizable spatio-temporal feature representations, enabling zero-shot and few-shot segmentation. SAM2 supports various prompts, including points, boxes, and masks, allowing users to specify targets flexibly and generate high-quality segmentation results. Unlike traditional single-frame image segmentation models, SAM2 can continuously track and segment objects in video sequences, achieving real-time inference with high accuracy. These capabilities make it particularly well-suited for applications that require low latency and high reliability, and its powerful generalization makes it an ideal starting point for adaptation to specific downstream medical tasks [11].

Semi-Supervised Learning (SSL) is a machine learning paradigm which bridges supervised and unsupervised learning. Its main idea is to leverage a small amount of labeled data together with a large amount of unlabeled data to train a model. This approach addresses the challenges of high annotation costs and the scarcity of labeled samples [12]. Among the various SSL methods, pseudo-labeling is widely adopted due to its simplicity and effectiveness. The core principle of this method is to first train a model on the available labeled data, and then use this model to generate predictions on the unlabeled data, which are used as "pseudo-labels" to augment the original labeled dataset. This process is often performed iteratively to progressively improve model performance [13].

This paper aims to efficiently adapt the high-performing SAM2 model from the general vision domain to the specific task of tumor segmentation in TrackRAD2025. We propose a novel three-stage semi-supervised fine-tuning framework. First, the framework systematically evaluates and screens the foundation model to select the optimal starting point. Second, it uses a limited amount of labeled data for supervised, full-parameter fine-tuning to learn domain-specific features. Finally, through pseudo-label generation and iterative self-training, it leverages large-scale unlabeled data to further enhance the model's accuracy and robustness. An overview of the proposed method is shown in Fig. 1.

Our core contributions include:

1. Designing a systematic fine-tuning approach that progresses from generalization to specialization, followed by data-driven reinforcement, addressing the challenge of limited labeled data in medical image segmentation.
2. Utilizing large-scale unlabeled data through a pseudo-label generation mechanism, enhancing the model's segmentation accuracy and robustness.
3. Validating the method on the TrackRAD2025 dataset, securing second place in the competition and offering a practical reference for the clinical application of foundation models in radiotherapy.

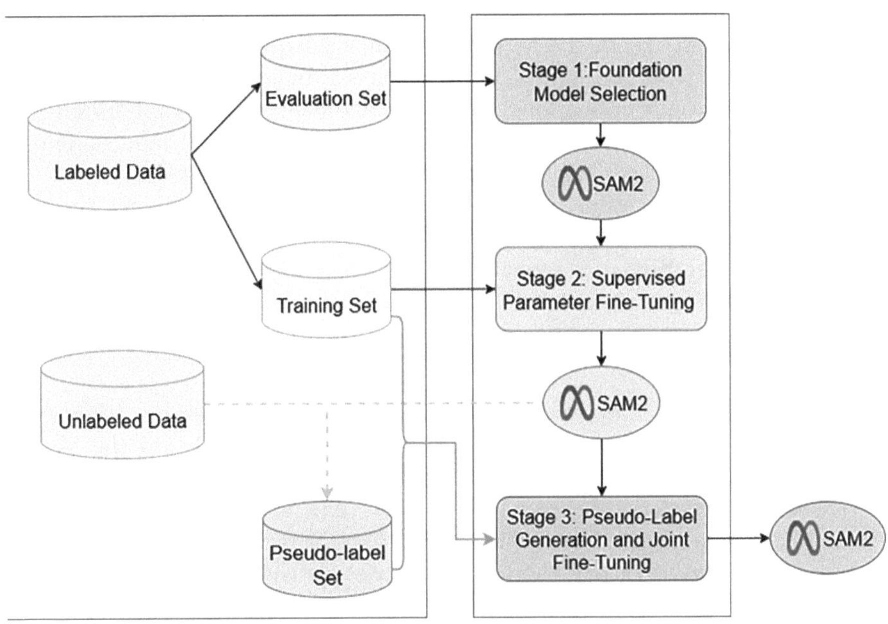

Fig. 1. Overview of the proposed three-stage semi-supervised fine-tuning method for real-time MRI tumor segmentation in TrackRAD2025. Stage 1 selects a foundation model based on SAM2. Stage 2 performs supervised parameter fine-tuning with the foundation model and generates pseudo-labels for unlabeled data. Stage 3 fine-tunes the model on the combined labeled and pseudo-labeled data to improve generalization.

Table 1. Data partition for the three-stage training and evaluation process.

Data Source (N)	Subset	Number	Purpose
Labeled data (50)	Evaluation set	12	Model performance evaluation
	Training Set	38	Supervised fine-tuning
Unlabeled data (477)	Pseudo-label Set	100	Pseudo-label generation and joint training

2 Method

2.1 Data

Dataset Partitioning. This study utilized exclusively data from the TrackRAD2025 challenge[1], which targets tumor tracking in time-resolved sagittal 2D cine-MRI sequences [14], without incorporating any external datasets. The dataset consists of 108 labeled sequences, including 50 publicly available sequences for training and 58 non-public sequences for validation, along with 477 unlabeled sequences. All images and their segmentation masks are stored in the `.mha` format.

To carry out the three-stage training and evaluation process proposed in this study, the dataset was systematically divided, as summarized in Table 1.

Evaluation Set: From the 50 publicly labeled sequences, 12 samples were selected through stratified sampling to ensure a balanced representation of data centers, anatomical locations, and magnetic field strengths. This set was employed in Stage 1 to evaluate and screen pre-trained SAM2 models, and it was also used for local performance assessment in subsequent stages.

Training Set: The remaining 38 publicly labeled sequences were assigned for Stage 2 full-parameter supervised fine-tuning.

Pseudo-Label Set: 100 sequences were selected from the 477 unlabeled sequences. Following pseudo-label generation, these samples were utilized for Stage 3 semi-supervised learning.

Data Processing. To leverage the existing training and inference framework of SAM2, the selected TrackRAD2025 dataset was converted into the MOSE dataset format [15]. Note that the MOSE dataset uses PNG images; accordingly, the TrackRAD2025 data were converted from `.mha` to PNG format to maintain consistency with the MOSE structure. Being a representative benchmark in video object segmentation, the MOSE dataset structure supports sequential inputs, per-frame annotations, and a consistent data representation. This format not only ensures strong compatibility with the SAM2 implementation but also provides several advantages:

(1) **Technical compatibility and training efficiency**: The MOSE format aligns with mainstream video object segmentation benchmarks, allowing direct reuse of existing SAM2 training pipelines and avoiding complex preprocessing.

[1] https://trackrad2025.grand-challenge.org/.

Unlike the original `.mha` format, which stores an entire video sequence in a single file and imposes memory constraints, the MOSE format enables per-frame or small-clip data access, facilitating multi-frame loading strategies and improving training efficiency. (2) **Cross-domain methodological transfer**: Tumor tracking in cine-MRI and video object segmentation share core temporal segmentation challenges such as object deformation, motion blur, and background interference. Adopting the MOSE format allows the transfer of advanced computer vision methods to medical imaging, thereby facilitating research and providing new insights. (3) **Enhanced reproducibility and standardization**: A standardized data format ensures transparent experimental setups and more consistent performance comparisons. Overall, this conversion is motivated by both technical and methodological considerations, improving the translatability and reproducibility of tumor tracking research across domains.

Pseudo-Label Generation for Semi-supervised Training. To generate high-quality pseudo-labels for the unlabeled cine-MRI data using SAM2, it was necessary to provide rectangular bounding box prompts. In the absence of expert annotations, we used the labeled data to identify characteristic tumor features—such as hypointense lesions, hyperintense rims, and round or oval shapes—across different magnetic field strengths (0.35T and 1.5T) and anatomical locations (pelvis, abdomen, and chest). Based on these observations, we manually estimated approximate tumor locations to construct the rectangular prompts for the unlabeled dataset. However, this manual, experience-based approach is subject to several uncertainties: (1) tissue contrast varies considerably across patients and MRI sequences, leading to heterogeneous tumor appearances; (2) the generated pseudo-label bounding boxes may be oversized or misaligned with the true tumor location, introducing noise.

Therefore, these pseudo-labels are regarded as weak supervision rather than precise ground truth. To mitigate this uncertainty, we optimized the subsequent semi-supervised training by adjusting the loss function weights and learning rate.

Dataset Characteristics. To evaluate and enhance the model's generalization ability, we performed a detailed analysis of dataset characteristics. Data diversity, especially across three key variables—data source center, anatomical location, and magnetic field strength—is essential for training models that can perform reliably on unseen data from diverse clinical environments. Models trained on homogeneous datasets often show degraded performance when applied to data from different centers or under varying imaging conditions. To address this, we used circular statistical charts 2 to visualize the proportional distribution of the dataset along these dimensions, with three objectives: (1) assessing cross-center generalization by analyzing data distribution across medical centers and identifying potential source-specific biases; (2) ensuring anatomical coverage by quantifying the proportions of pelvis, abdomen, and thorax data, thereby improving lesion identification across regions; (3) considering magnetic field strength by comparing proportions at 0.35T and 1.5T, thus assessing robustness to imaging equipment variability.

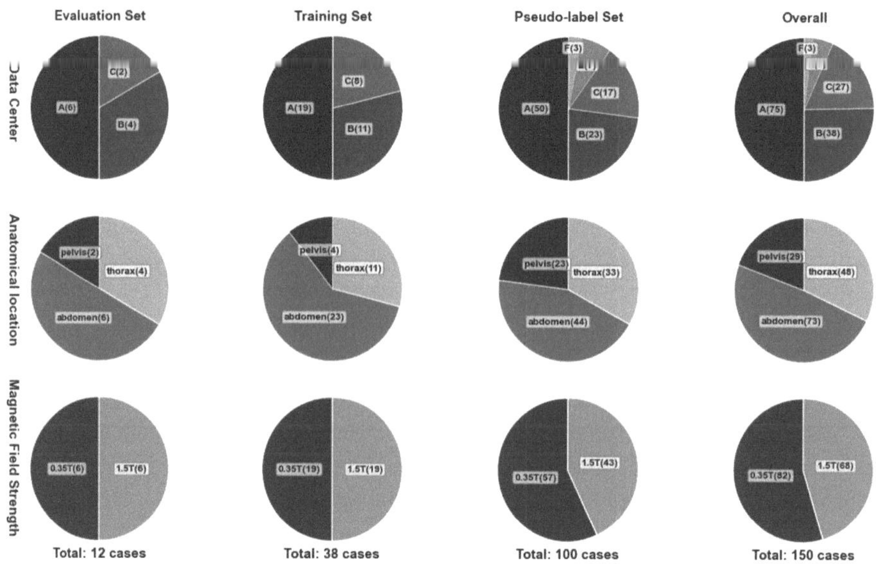

Fig. 2. Circular charts illustrating the dataset distribution across medical centers, anatomical locations, magnetic field strengths, and their overall composition.

2.2 Model

SAM2 was selected as the backbone segmentation model for the tumor segmentation task on cine-MRI sequences. As a foundation model, SAM2 is designed for promptable segmentation of images and videos (as shown in Fig. 3). The model consists of three core components: (1) an **Image Encoder** that extracts visual features from image or video frames, (2) a **Prompt Encoder** that converts various prompts (e.g., points, boxes, and masks) into a unified vector representation, and (3) a **Mask Decoder** that integrates the visual features with the prompt embeddings to generate the final segmentation outputs [11]. The Image Encoder is built upon Hiera [17], a hierarchical vision transformer pre-trained with Masked Autoencoding (MAE) [18]. It efficiently extracts rich hierarchical features from complex scenes, and its performance is crucial for the model's overall segmentation accuracy and generalization.

The core advantage of SAM2 lies in its innovative streaming memory module for video processing. This module employs both self-attention and cross-attention to integrate temporal information from past frames into current-frame segmentation. By conditioning inference on historical context, the model achieves improved temporal coherence while maintaining real-time performance. This

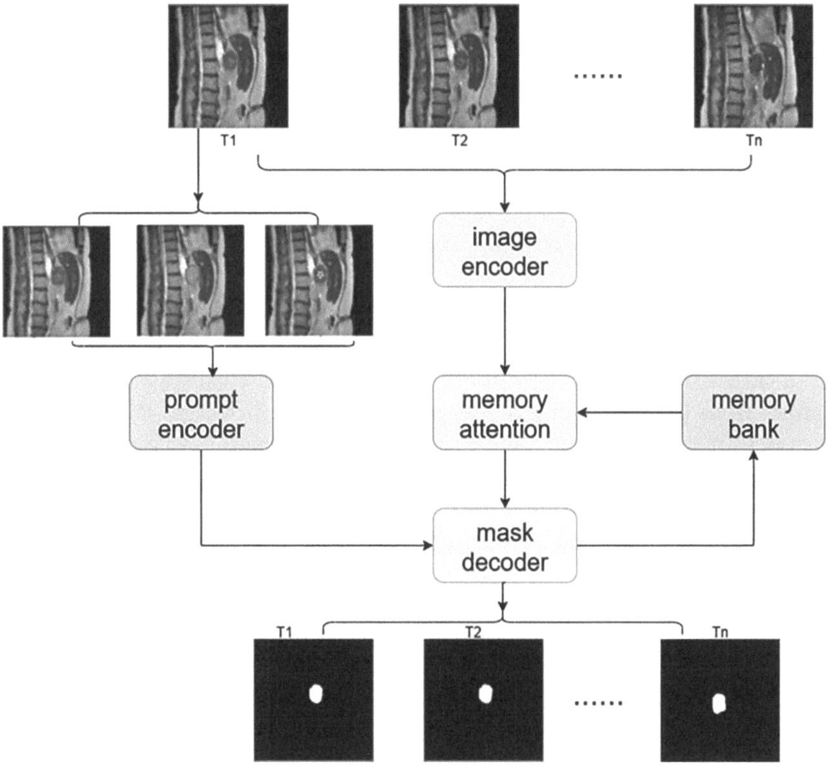

Fig. 3. Illustration of the SAM2 architecture, showing the image encoder, prompt encoder, and mask decoder. During both training and evaluation, the model receives boxes, points, and masks from the first frame as input prompts.

mechanism is a primary factor underlying SAM2's superior performance compared to its predecessor [19].

In the first stage of our approach, we selected a foundation model for tumor segmentation. We employed the tumor mask, bounding box, and center point as prompts (as shown in Fig. 3), and chose `sam2.1_hiera_tiny` as the core model. This choice was motivated by its relatively small parameter size—38.9M compared to 224.4M in `sam2.1_hiera_large`—while still retaining the multi-scale feature representation capability of the Hiera Transformer. These characteristics make it particularly suitable for fine-tuning on small-sample medical datasets, thereby improving both training stability and generalization.

The model parameters were initialized using official pre-trained weights. Specifically, the weights of the image encoder, prompt encoder, and mask decoder were loaded from the pre-trained checkpoints and fine-tuned, instead of random initialization. The model was adapted to the cine-MRI tumor segmentation task through a combination of supervised training on labeled data and semi-supervised training on unlabeled data. The entire framework was implemented in PyTorch, with supporting libraries such as `SimpleITK`, `NumPy`, `iopath`, `hydra-core`, `Matplotlib`, `CSV`, and `Pandas` for data processing, visualization, and configuration management. Training was conducted on a workstation equipped with an NVIDIA GeForce RTX 3090 GPU (24GB), an Intel Core i5-12490F CPU (12th Gen), and 32GB RAM, running CUDA 12.4. To ensure reproducibility, we relied on the official SAM2 repository on GitHub[2], which provides inference code, checkpoint download links, and example notebooks.

2.3 Training

To better leverage SAM2's generalization capability for our specific task, we designed a three-stage progressive fine-tuning strategy. In each stage, the following prompts from the first frame were used as model inputs: (1) the bounding box corresponding to the tumor mask, (2) the central point within the mask, and (3) the mask itself.

During training, the batch size was set to 2 and training was run for 200 epochs. We employed the AdamW optimizer, which is well-suited for fine-tuning large models with effective weight decay regularization. A cosine decay learning rate scheduler was applied, which starts with a high learning rate for rapid convergence and gradually decreases it to improve precision and mitigate overfitting.

Data augmentation followed the official SAM2 training pipeline, including geometric transformations (flipping, affine transformations, and random scaling to 512×512) along with color augmentations (random brightness, contrast, saturation, and grayscale). All images were normalized by applying a linear intensity rescaling within each frame, mapping the minimum and maximum pixel values to 0 and 255, respectively, and subsequently converted to 8-bit unsigned integer (uint8) format to ensure consistency and compatibility with standard image processing pipelines. The following sections describe each of the three training stages in detail.

Stage One: Foundation Model Evaluation and Selection. In the first stage, we sought to identify the optimal zero-shot model on the TrackRAD2025 dataset among several official SAM2 pre-trained variants. We used the official evaluation code provided by the challenge to assess four models-`sam2.1_hiera_tiny`, `sam2_hiera_small`, `sam2_hiera_base_plus`, and `sam2_hiera_large` on a dedicated evaluation set. Based on experimental results and theoretical analysis, the best-performing foundation model was selected for the subsequent stage of training.

Stage Two: Supervised Parameter Fine-Tuning. The objective of this stage was to fine-tune the pre-trained model selected in Stage One on the supervised training set. This process adapts the model's general segmentation capa-

[2] https://github.com/facebookresearch/sam2.

bilities for cine-MRI tumor segmentation, thereby improving segmentation accuracy on small-sample medical datasets. We compared the fine-tuning results of different model modules to identify the most effective strategy for subsequent pseudo-label generation in Stage Three.

Training samples from the supervised dataset were randomly presented with either a bounding box or a central point prompt with 50 % probability to enhance robustness to different prompt types. We adopted the multi-task loss function from the official SAM2 training code, which includes mask loss, Dice loss, IoU loss, and class loss, with weights set according to the default values in the official SAM2 training template. The relatively higher weight of the mask loss, as defined in the template, ensures high segmentation accuracy while preserving overall prediction consistency and class information.

A cosine decay learning rate scheduler was applied, with a global learning rate decaying from 2.0×10^{-7} to 2.0×10^{-8}. A lower learning rate was applied to the image encoder, decaying from 1.0×10^{-7} to 1.0×10^{-8}.

Stage Three: Pseudo-Label Generation and Joint Fine-Tuning. To address the limited size of the annotated dataset, we adopted a semi-supervised pseudo-label learning strategy to further improve the model's performance and generalization by leveraging unlabeled data. The optimal model from Stage Two's supervised fine-tuning was first used to perform inference on the unlabeled data. A bounding box was used as the sole prompt to generate tumor segmentation masks, which served as pseudo-labels.

The supervised and semi-supervised datasets were then combined to form a total of 138 sequences. This approach offered two key benefits: (1) maximizing data utilization by incorporating valuable unlabeled information, and (2) enhancing model generalization by mitigating the impact of pseudo-label noise on performance.

The best-performing model from Stage Two was subsequently fine-tuned on the combined dataset. This allowed us to take advantage of the increased sample size provided by pseudo-labels to enhance the model's generalization across centers, anatomical regions, and magnetic field strengths. During this final fine-tuning stage, the same loss function and fine-tuning parameters from Stage Two were used, with adjusted loss weights and learning rate to better utilize pseudo-labels during model optimization.

2.4 Evaluation

To ensure fair, consistent, and comparable evaluation across studies, we adhered to the official TrackRAD2025 challenge guidelines. All performance metrics were computed using the standardized evaluation code provided by the organizers, applied to the evaluation set described in Sect. 2.1.

The evaluation framework covers four key dimensions: segmentation accuracy, geometric consistency, clinical relevance, and operational efficiency. The specific metrics are summarized in Table 2.

Table 2. Overview of evaluation metrics for the TrackRAD2025 challenge.

Category	Metric	Description	Unit	Target
Segmentation Accuracy	Dice Similarity Coefficient (DSC)	Volumetric overlap between prediction and ground truth	Unitless	≈ 1
	Hausdorff Distance 95 (HD95)	Maximum boundary deviation at the 95th percentile	Pixels	minimize
	Average Surface Distance (ASD)	Mean surface distance reflecting boundary fit	Pixels	minimize
Geometric Consistency	Center Distance (CD)	Euclidean distance between predicted and true centers	Pixels	minimize
Clinical Relevance	Relative D98 Dose (D98)	Minimum dose to 98% of the predicted target volume relative to ground truth	Unitless	≈ 1
Operational Efficiency	Runtime (RT)	Mean inference time per case, excluding model loading and data preparation	Seconds(s)	minimize
	Loading Time (LT)	Estimated time required for model initialization and data preprocessing, shared across all cases	Seconds(s)	minimize
	Time Per Frame (TPF)	Time to process a single frame	Seconds(s)	minimize
	Total Time (TT)	Sum of all elapsed times for the complete workflow, including loading, preprocessing, and inference	Seconds(s)	minimize

3 Results

At each stage of model development, we conduct a systematic analysis of model performance using the evaluation metrics presented in Sect. 2.4. All results, presented in tables and text, strictly follow the units specified in the same section, ensuring consistency and enabling accurate comparisons across experiments. This analysis provides a solid foundation for selecting the best-performing model and refining it further.

3.1 Stage One Results

In the first stage, we evaluate the zero-shot performance of four pre-trained SAM2 models on our evaluation set to identify the foundation model with the highest zero-shot performance. The evaluation results are summarized in Table 3.

Table 3. SAM2 Foundation Model Performance Evaluation. Best values for each metric are highlighted in **bold**.

Foundation Model	DSC↑	HD95↓	ASD↓	CD↓	D98↑	RT↓	LT↓	TPF↓	TT↓
`sam2.1_hiera_tiny`	0.8912	3.3827	1.2462	1.4555	0.9236	**8.7336**	4.3390	**0.0746**	**156.87**
`sam2.1_hiera_small`	**0.8923**	3.3505	1.2352	1.4686	0.9087	12.761	**2.2039**	0.1089	179.57
`sam2.1_hiera_large`	0.8917	**3.2958**	1.2373	**1.3838**	**0.9266**	15.275	5.0446	0.1305	243.83
`sam2.1_hiera_base_plus`	0.8901	3.3881	**1.2243**	1.3923	0.9171	12.009	3.0845	0.1026	181.12

The results of the initial evaluation demonstrate that the tiny model, while maintaining high segmentation accuracy, achieves faster inference speed compared to the other variants. Specifically, its Dice coefficient of 0.8912 is highly competitive with those of the small (0.8923) and large (0.8917) models, differing by less than 0.2 %. Moreover, its average per-frame inference time is

0.075 s/frame, corresponding to a 31 %-42 % speedup relative to the small and large models.

Furthermore, although the dosimetric indicators of the tiny model are slightly lower than those of the large model, they remain clinically acceptable, supporting its reliability for clinical application. In real-time tumor tracking, low-latency inference is critical for practical usability, as the system must rapidly respond to changes in tumor location and morphology. Excessive computational overhead can lead to tracking delays, potentially compromising treatment accuracy and patient safety.

While the large model performs best on some boundary and dosimetric metrics, the tiny model provides the best balance between speed and accuracy. It achieves a significant speed advantage with minimal loss in segmentation performance. Therefore, we selected the tiny model as the foundation for subsequent fine-tuning to satisfy the performance requirements of the TrackRAD2025 challenge in real-time tumor tracking.

3.2 Stage Two Results

In this stage, we fine-tune the `sam2.1_hiera_tiny` base model through experiments with different parameter-tuning modules to determine the most effective strategy. Experimental results are summarized in Table 4.

Table 4. Performance of different fine-tuning modules in Stage Two. Best values for each metric are highlighted in **bold**.

Fine-tuning Module	DSC↑	HD95↓	ASD↓	CD↓	D98↑	RT↓	LT↓	TPF↓	TT↓
Full Parameters	**0.9001**	**3.1465**	**1.1605**	**1.3339**	0.9239	8.2026	4.7309	0.0701	155.20
Mask	0.8907	3.3117	1.2016	1.4325	0.9242	8.6775	8.6776	0.0741	158.28
Prompt	0.8925	3.3190	1.2298	1.4239	**0.9297**	**8.0214**	**4.5643**	**0.0685**	**151.03**
Mask+Prompt	0.8908	3.3120	1.2016	1.4331	0.9186	8.8949	4.2124	0.0759	157.29

A comparison of the four fine-tuning strategies reveals notable differences in their segmentation performance and efficiency. First, in terms of geometric consistency, full-parameter fine-tuning yields the best results across all key metrics. It achieves the highest DSC (0.9001), significantly outperforming both mask and prompt-based methods. The 95 % Hausdorff Distance and Average Surface Distance of full-parameter fine-tuning are reduced to 3.146 and 1.160, respectively. These results indicate that full-parameter fine-tuning is most effective in preserving both the morphological consistency and spatial localization accuracy of the tumor.

Regarding the clinically relevant Relative D98 metric, prompt fine-tuning demonstrates a marginal advantage over full-parameter fine-tuning (0.930 vs. 0.924). However, this limited difference is insufficient to outweigh the significant gains in geometric accuracy, which are provided by full-parameter fine-tuning.

While prompt fine-tuning has a slight edge in overall runtime, the overall time difference is less than 5 %. This minimal variance suggests that the efficiency of full-parameter fine-tuning is sufficient for practical applications.

In conclusion, our analysis shows that full-parameter fine-tuning is the most effective strategy under our experimental conditions. It not only achieves superior segmentation performance but also maintains a high level of operational efficiency, thereby significantly enhancing both the geometric accuracy and clinical applicability of the model.

3.3 Stage Three Results

This stage focuses on semi-supervised training on the combined dataset. We optimize the model through adjustment of key hyperparameters, including learning rate and loss function weights, to determine the best-performing model. The experimental results are presented in Table 5.

Table 5. Hyperparameter tuning results for Stage Three.

Hyperparameter	DSC↑	HD95↓	ASD↓	CD↓	D98↑	RT↓	LT↓	TPF↓	**TT↓**
base_lr = 2.0e-06, mask = 20, dice = 5, iou = 1, class = 1	0.9047	3.0520	1.1078	1.3539	0.9319	9.9220	3.5194	0.0847	161.29
base_lr = 2.0e-07, mask = 30, dice = 1, iou = 1, class = 1	0.9039	3.0637	1.1151	1.2679	**0.9412**	10.767	**3.0097**	0.0919	165.32
base_lr = 2.0e-07, mask = 10, dice = 5, iou = 20, class = 1	0.9048	3.0119	1.0956	1.2463	0.9383	9.1420	4.0983	0.0781	158.88
base_lr = 2.0e-07, mask = 1, dice = 40, iou = 1, class = 1	**0.9073**	2.9441	**1.0676**	1.2785	0.9267	8.7628	5.0899	0.0748	166.23
base_lr = 2.0e-07, mask = 1, dice = 10, iou = 30, class = 1	**0.9073**	**2.9239**	1.0695	**1.2328**	0.9398	**8.9995**	4.2021	0.0768	**158.42**

Our experimental results indicate that different configurations of loss function weights and learning rate schedules have varied effects on model performance. Compared to the baseline full-parameter fine-tuning, configurations with a lower learning rate and higher weights for Dice and IoU losses (rows 4 and 5 in Table 5) demonstrate superior segmentation accuracy.

Specifically, the fourth configuration achieves the best results in both Dice Similarity Coefficient and Average Surface Distance, excelling in overall segmentation performance. The fifth configuration, however, significantly outperforms other methods in 95 % Hausdorff Distance and Center Distance, highlighting its geometric accuracy and boundary precision.

Consequently, we conclude that the fourth and fifth configurations represent the most effective solutions under our experimental conditions. Both effectively improve boundary fitting and spatial consistency while maintaining high overall segmentation accuracy. The choice between them depends on the specific task requirements: the fifth configuration is better suited for tasks prioritizing geometric precision and boundary accuracy, whereas the fourth configuration is advantageous when the focus is on global segmentation performance and average surface consistency.

For our final submission to the TrackRAD2025 challenge, we selected the model trained with the fifth configuration.

4 Discussion

In this study, we successfully adapt the SAM2 model for the complex task of real-time MRI tumor tracking. Our proposed three-stage incremental fine-tuning strategy proves to be highly effective. The experimental results demonstrate its success in leveraging the power of a foundation model for a specialized medical application.

Our primary contribution is the development and validation of a progressive "selection-supervised-semi-supervised" learning pipeline, which maximizes the potential of a large-scale foundation model. Notably, the introduction of pseudo-label enhanced training in the third stage effectively utilizes a large volume of unlabeled data. This approach significantly reduces our dependence on extensive manual annotations and ultimately enhances the model's generalization capabilities.

Despite our strong results, our method still has several limitations. First, the quality of the pseudo-labels is directly dependent on the performance of the Stage Two model. This presents a risk of "confirmation bias," where the model may reinforce its own potential errors. It is crucial to note that the bounding box prompts used for pseudo-label generation are derived from manual, rule-based inference rather than expert annotations, rendering their accuracy uncertain. Consequently, these pseudo-labels are best viewed as a weak supervision signal rather than a gold standard. Second, the model's segmentation boundaries for images with extremely low contrast remain inconsistent, indicating the need for further refinement.

Author contributions. Kailin He: Writing – review & editing, Writing – original draft, Visualization, Validation, Software, Methodology, Formal analysis, Data curation, Conceptualization. **Shengqian Zhu:** Writing – review & editing. **Ying Song:** Writing – review & editing, Supervision, Resources, Funding acquisition. **Guangjun Li:** Writing – review & editing, Supervision, Resources, Funding acquisition. **Junjie Hu:** Writing – review & editing, Supervision, Resources, Funding acquisition.

Other information. This work was supported by the National Natural Science Foundation of China under Grant 62476184, Natural Science Foundation from the Science and Technology Department of Sichuan Province under Grant 2024NSFTD0051 and 2024NSFSC1789.

References

1. Otazo, R., et al.: MRI-guided radiation therapy: an emerging paradigm in adaptive radiation oncology. Radiology **298**(2), 248–260 (2021)
2. Keall, P.J., et al.: Integrated MRI-guided radiotherapy - opportunities and challenges. Nat. Rev. Clin. Oncol. **19**(7), 458–470 (2022)
3. Kurz, C., et al.: Medical physics challenges in clinical MR-guided radiotherapy. Radiat. Oncol. **15**, 93 (2020)
4. Salari, E., Wang, J., Wynne, J.F., Chang, C.W., Wu, Y., Yang, X.: Artificial intelligence-based motion tracking in cancer radiotherapy: a review. J. Appl. Clin. Med. Phys. **25**(11), e14500 (2024)
5. Muren, L.P.: Physics and imaging in radiation oncology comes of age. Phys. Imaging Radiat. Oncol. **29**, 100559 (2024)
6. Bommasani, R.: On the opportunities and risks of foundation models. arXiv preprint: arXiv:2108.07258 (2021)
7. Awais, M., et al.: Foundation models defining a new era in vision: a survey and outlook. IEEE Trans. Pattern Anal. Mach. Intell. **47**(4), 2245–2264 (2025)
8. Schneider, J.: Foundation models in brief: a historical, socio-technical focus. arXiv preprint: arXiv:2212.08967 (2022)
9. Chia, M.A., Antaki, F., Zhou, Y., Turner, A.W., Lee, A.Y., Keane, P.A.: Foundation models in ophthalmology. Br. J. Ophthalmol. **108**(10), 1341–1348 (2024)
10. Li, J.: Large language models and foundation models in smart agriculture: basics, opportunities, and challenges. arXiv preprint: arXiv:2308.06668 (2023)
11. Ravi, N.: SAM 2: segment anything in images and videos. arXiv preprint: arXiv:2408.00714 (2024)
12. Jiao, R., et al.: Learning with limited annotations: a survey on deep semi-supervised learning for medical image segmentation. Comput. Biol. Med. **169**, 107840 (2024)
13. Ran, L., Li, Y., Liang, G., Zhang, Y.: Pseudo labeling methods for semi-supervised semantic segmentation: a review and future perspectives. IEEE Trans. Circuits Syst. Video Technol. **35**(4), 3054–3080 (2025)
14. Wang, Y.: TrackRAD2025 challenge dataset: real-time tumor tracking for MRI-guided radiotherapy. arXiv preprint: arXiv:2503.19119 (2025)
15. Ding, H., Liu, C., He, S., Jiang, X., Torr, P.H.S., Bai, S.: MOSE: a new dataset for video object segmentation in complex scenes. arXiv preprint: arXiv:2302.01872 (2023)
16. Xu, N.: YouTube-VOS: sequence-to-sequence video object segmentation. arXiv preprint: arXiv:1809.00461 (2018)
17. Ryali, C., et al.: Hiera: a hierarchical vision transformer without the bells-and-whistles. In: Proceedings of the PMLR, pp. 29441–29454 (2023)
18. He, K., Chen, X., Xie, S., Li, Y., Dollár, P., Girshick, R.: Masked autoencoders are scalable vision learners. In: Proceedings of the Conference, pp. 16000–16009 (2022)
19. Xu, G., Kabat, C., Zhang, Y.: Depthwise-dilated convolutional adapters for medical object tracking and segmentation using the Segment Anything Model 2. arXiv preprint: arXiv:2507.14613 (2025)

Tumor Tracking as Point Tracking: CoTracker3 in the TrackRAD2025 Challenge

Felix Knispel[1,2](✉) and Sergios Gatidis[2]

[1] RWTH Aachen University, Aachen, Germany
felix.knispel@rwth-aachen.de
[2] Stanford University, Stanford, CA, USA

Abstract. The TrackRAD2025 challenge provides a common benchmark dataset and evaluation framework for algorithms to improve real-time tumor tracking in the context of MRI-guided radiotherapy.

In this work, we propose to reframe segmentation mask tracking as boundary point tracking and evaluate the effectiveness of the pre-trained CoTracker3 model [2]. We introduce a method to convert between segmentation masks and boundary points and vice versa, enabling the use of any pre-trained point tracking model for segmentation mask tracking.

Our submission to the TrackRAD2025 challenge does not require any cine-MRI data for training nor fine-tuning of models. Evaluation is performed as part of the TrackRAD2025 evaluation framework on both publicly available and held-out data. Our submission ranked third place on the challenge leaderboard and shows robust performance across held-out datasets and data acquisition sites. We demonstrate that off-the-shelf point tracking models trained on natural videos can transfer effectively to real-time tumor tracking for MRI-guided radiotherapy without any labeled data or computationally expensive training.

1 Introduction

1.1 Background and Motivation

The TrackRAD2025 challenge calls for improved methods for real-time tumor tracking in the context of MRI-guided radiotherapy. Organizers provide a large, multi-centric labeled and unlabeled dataset along with a unified evaluation framework [11].

Existing and conventional registration-based techniques used in adaptive radiotherapy often struggle with non-rigid motion and image variability across scanners, motivating deep learning-based alternatives. Increased accuracy, robustness, and real-time applicability promise more efficient radiation delivery, potentially reducing treatment duration and enabling higher patient throughput.

A widespread limitation in medical image analysis is the scarcity of high-quality labeled data. While TrackRAD supplies a curated labeled dataset, its scale is relatively small compared to the requirements of modern deep learning

J. P. Wachs et al. (Eds.): TrackRAD/TTC 2025, LNCS 16474, pp. 17–24, 2027.
https://doi.org/10.1007/978-3-032-35046-6_2

systems with millions of trainable parameters. Achieving robust performance in clinical deployment requires diverse training data spanning multiple sites, scanners, imaging protocols, and patient populations.

Strategies to mitigate the issue of data scarcity oftentimes involve forms of self-supervised learning, synthetic augmentation, or pseudo-labeling. Alternatively, pre-trained, general-purpose foundation models - originally trained on primarily non-medical data - have shown surprising transferability to tasks across the medical domain.

In this work, we investigate whether a state-of-the-art point tracking model originally trained on natural videos can perform tumor tracking without any domain-specific training or fine-tuning.

1.2 Tracking Any Point (TAP)

The TrackRAD challenge presents a tumor tracking task, which can be interpreted as a "segmentation mask tracking through time" task. Popular pre-trained foundation models for such tasks include the Segment Anything (SAM) model family [4].

A highly related problem in computer vision is the task of *Tracking Any Point* (TAP): Given a sequence of images as well as a set of query points in a single frame, TAP models are tasked with predicting precise trajectories of queried points throughout the entire sequence of images. Recent TAP models such as TAPIR [1], CoTracker [3], or CoTracker3 [2] are able to track thousands of points through long video sequences. These models can track points through occlusions and support real-time inference in online prediction settings.

The issue of labeled data being scarce in this field has been addressed through e.g. a large synthetically generated, exactly-labeled dataset or pseudolabeling techniques [2] (Fig. 1).

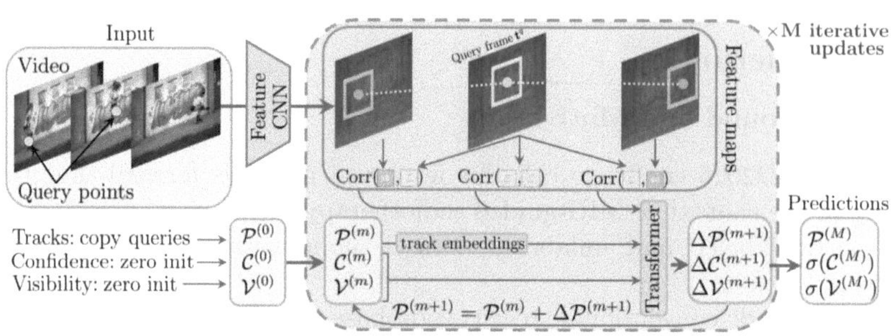

Fig. 1. Schema: CoTracker Architecture Taken from [2]. Tracks are updated iteratively based on the correlation of CNN-extracted features at estimated point locations across timesteps.

CoTracker3. The CoTracker3 model as introduced in [2] is considered a state-of-the-art point tracking model for natural video sequences.

Its architecture uses a CNN to extract feature maps around tracked points from each input video frame at multiple scales. Correlation of feature maps between query and target frames is computed into a single 4D correlation volume. This volume's dimensionality is then reduced by projecting it into a lower-dimensional space using a MLP. Lastly, a transformer component iteratively refines predictions of point displacement, point visibility and prediction confidence. This transformer uses attention over both time and across tracked points ("tracks").

An interesting aspect of the CoTracker3 architecture is the training scheme proposed by Karaev et al., which combines a large-scale synthetic dataset with the *pseudo-labeling* of real-world data to bridge the gap between the synthetic and real-world data domains. Initially, several *teacher models* are pre-trained on a synthetically generated dataset, where exact labels are obtained directly from the data generation process. A *student model*, which is initially pre-trained on this synthetic dataset as well, is then fine-tuned on real-world video data. The real-world video data however does not come with any labels. Instead, the teacher models are used to "pseudo-label" the real-world video data on the fly.

Although the teacher-provided label are considered noisy and suboptimal, they enable the student model to adapt to the real-world data domain and improve performance on point-tracking benchmarks. We refer to [2] for further details on the architecture and training process.

2 Methods

We investigate the capabilities of CoTracker3 [2], a point tracking model trained on natural videos, for the task of tumor tracking in MRI sequences. We propose to reframe the segmentation mask tracking problem as a point correspondence task by converting segmentation mask boundaries to tracked points and vice versa. This allows us to make use of a pre-trained CoTracker3 instance without any training of our own.

The code used to participate in the TrackRAD2025 challenge can be found at https://github.com/felixknispel/trackrad-cotracker-submission.

2.1 Data

For evaluation purposes, we considered only the provided TrackRAD2025 challenge data [11], specifically the 50 labeled cases from the training set. The labeled subset was used exclusively to validate: (1) the robustness of our bidirectional segmentation-to-points mapping technique, and (2) the performance of the pre-trained CoTracker3 model on medical imaging data. No training or hyperparameter optimization was performed. The unlabeled subset of the TrackRAD dataset was not utilized in our approach.

Converting from Masks to Points. We convert segmentation masks to sets of boundary points by sampling points along the outer boundary (or "contour") of the mask.

The `scikit-image` package's `measure.find_contours(...)` method [8] is used to obtain point coordinates of the contour of a given 2-dimensional segmentation mask. We subsequently sample n points from the set of contour points: After fitting a parametric spline to the irregular contour using the `scipy`-provided `splprep` function, we resample n evenly-spaced points using the `scipy.splev` function [9]. For this submission, we convert segmentation masks into point-based contours featuring $n = 1000$ points for each sample.

Recovering Masks from Points. After inference of the point tracking model, we need to recover the segmentation mask that is defined by the tracked points at their new locations. We make use of the OpenCV `fillPoly` method [7], which computes a filled polygon based on the provided sets of points.

The conversion process from segmentation masks to points and back to segmentation masks is effectively lossless (Fig. 2).

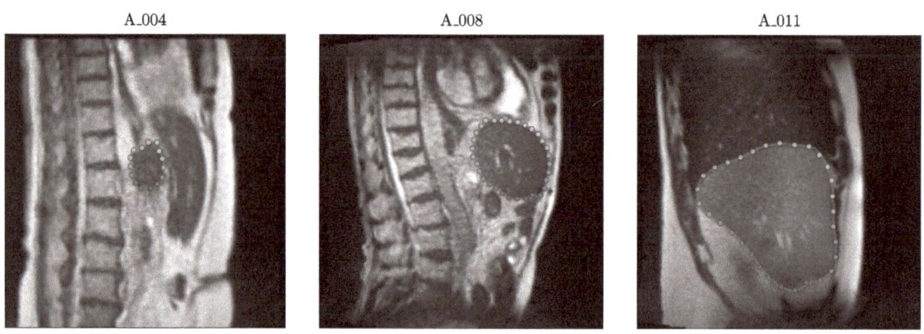

Fig. 2. Conversion examples: We compute an arbitrary number of boundary points for three samples from the TrackRAD2025 dataset and visualize them here. The red mask corresponds to the provided segmentation label. The colored points along the segmentation mask boundary represent the extracted points. These points are tracked as part of the CoTracker inference step to follow the movement in the underlying video sequence. For visualization purposes, we only display a subset of all extracted points. (Color figure online)

2.2 Tumor Tracking

We use the CoTracker3 model as defined and implemented in [2,5] without modification. Pre-trained weights of the `cotracker3_offline` model are available at Hugging Face [6] and used in this submission. We did not perform any hyperparameter optimization or training procedure to optimize the parameters or weights of the `cotracker3_offline` model.

Inference. We resize the cine-MRI images to size 384×512 pixels, as the pre-trained CoTracker3 model is configured to only work with videos of this shape. Inputs to the model are converted from the TrackRAD dataset using the method described in Sect. 2.1. Similar to Karaev et al. [2,3], we add a support grid of points to track during inference. Inference is performed in a single forward pass with the entire sequence loaded into memory. Visibility and confidence values output by the model are ignored, and support grid points are removed from the output. Coordinates are converted into the corresponding segmentation mask (as in Sect. 2.1) and resized back to the original image size.

2.3 Evaluation

To quantitatively evaluate the performance of our approach, we use the same metrics defined as the target endpoints of the challenge:

- Dice similarity coefficient ("Dice Coefficient")
- 95th percentile of the surface distance distribution ("Hausdorff 95%")
- The mean average surface distance ("Avg Surface Distance")
- Euclidean 2D center-of-mass error ("Center Distance")
- Relative simulated GTV D98% dose ("Relative D98 Dose")

We use the implementations provided in the official challenge repository [10]. We perform evaluation using the challenge-provided evaluation scripts & containers.

3 Results

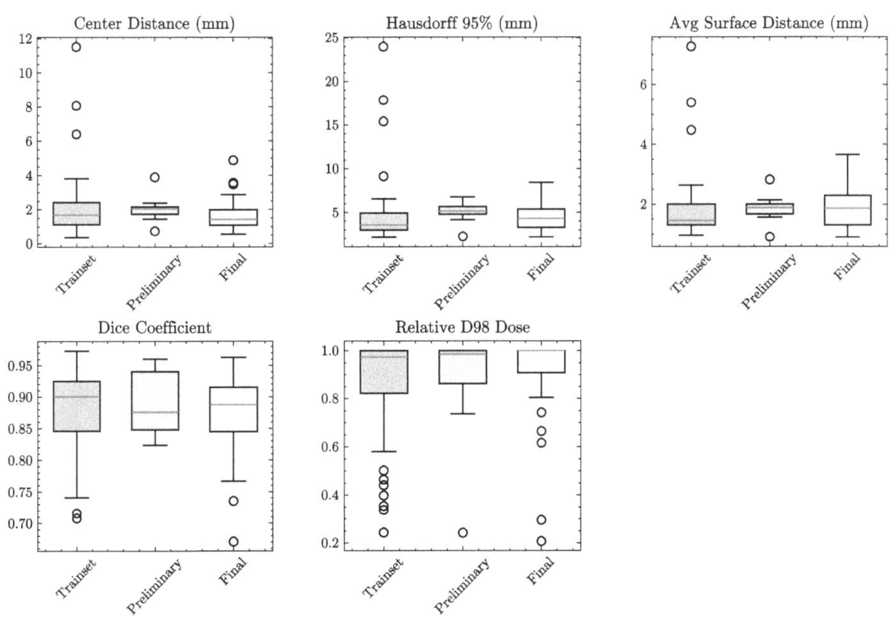

Fig. 3. Average performance metrics split by evaluation dataset: 50 labeled samples in training, 8 samples for preliminary testing, and 50 samples for final testing.

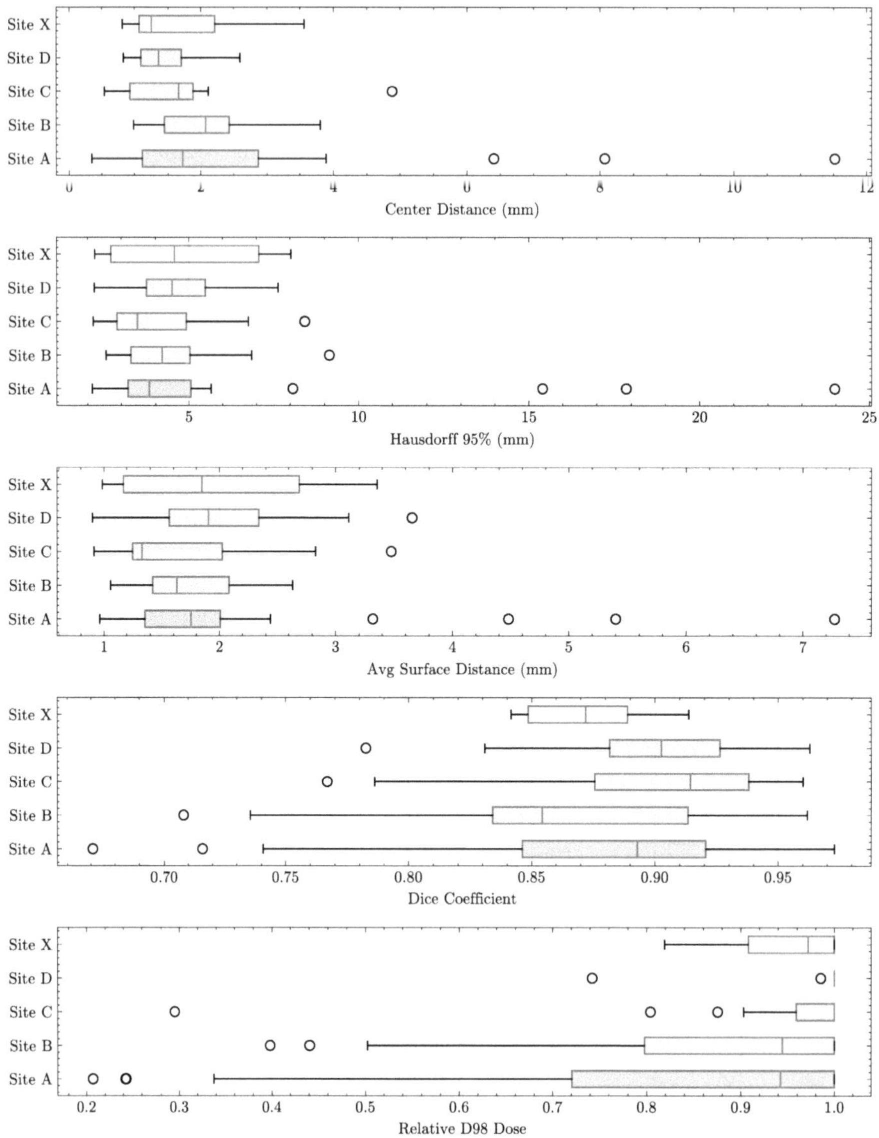

Fig. 4. Measured performance split by sample acquisition site.

We plot aggregate statistics over metrics across different datasets in Fig. 3 and across data acquisition sites in Fig. 4.

Manual inspection of numerous CoTracker3-provided predictions paints a picture of robustly tracked tumor masks. In areas of low contrast, such as in the lung, the model's predictions tend to differ from provided labels.

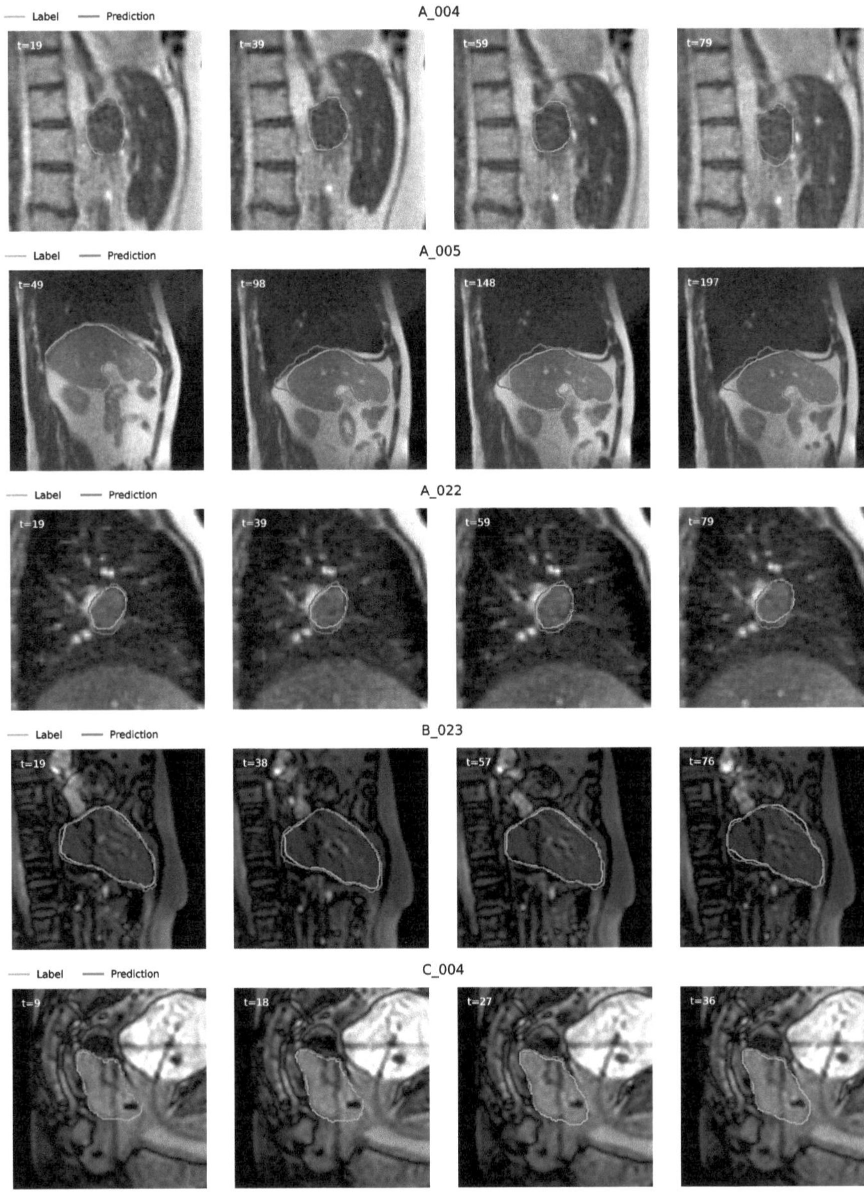

Fig. 5. CoTracker3 predictions vs. ground truth labels. Sampled at 4 time steps.

On our hardware (AMD EPYC 9654, NVIDIA RTX 6000 Ada), we find that inference of our method over a single TrackRAD sample takes around three to seven seconds, depending on the number of frames of the sample. This includes the loading of model weights from disk, which is usually performed in around 0.5–0.8 s on our hardware. The evaluation script reported an average runtime per frame of 0.017 on the training data set. The challenge algorithm evaluation system reported an average runtime per frame of 0.018 on the final test set and 0.100 on the preliminary test set (see Fig. 5).

4 Conclusion

We have introduced a method to convert between segmentation tracking and point tracking tasks, enabling the use of any pre-trained point tracking model for segmentation tracking. Our results utilizing the pre-trained CoTracker3 model demonstrate that point tracking models trained on natural videos can successfully track tumors in cine-MRI data without any domain-specific training or fine-tuning of the model.

Ongoing and future work investigates the potential of fine-tuning the CoTracker3 model to this challenge dataset and medical images in general.

Author contributions. FK: Conceptualization, Data Curation, Formal Analysis, Investigation, Methodology, Software, Validation, Visualization, Writing. SG: Conceptualization, Project Administration, Resources, Supervision.

References

1. Doersch, C., et al.: TAPIR: tracking any point with per-frame initialization and temporal refinement. In: Proceedings of the IEEE/CVF International Conference on Computer Vision, pp. 10061–10072 (2023)
2. Karaev, N., Makarov, I., Wang, J., Neverova, N., Vedaldi, A., Rupprecht, C.: CoTracker3: simpler and better point tracking by pseudo-labelling real videos. arXiv preprint: arXiv:2410.11831 (2024)
3. Karaev, N., Rocco, I., Graham, B., Neverova, N., Vedaldi, A., Rupprecht, C.: CoTracker: it is better to track together. In: Proceedings of the ECCV (2024)
4. Ma, J., et al.: MedSAM2: segment anything in 3D medical images and videos. arXiv preprint: arXiv:2504.03600 (2025)
5. Meta Research: GitHub – CoTracker3: simpler and better point tracking by pseudo-labelling real videos. https://github.com/facebookresearch/co-tracker
6. Meta Research: Hugging face – point tracking with CoTracker3. https://huggingface.co/facebook/cotracker3
7. Open Source Computer Vision Library: OpenCV Documentation – fillPoly. https://docs.opencv.org/4.x/d6/d6e/group__imgproc__draw.html#ga8c69b68fab5f25e2223b6496aa60dad5
8. The scikit-image team: scikit-image Documentation – skimage.measure.find_contours. https://scikit-image.org/docs/0.25.x/api/skimage.measure.html#skimage.measure.find_contours
9. The SciPy community: SciPy documentation – scipy.interpolate. https://docs.scipy.org/doc/scipy/reference/interpolate.html
10. The TrackRAD2025 organizers: Trackrad 2025. https://github.com/LMUK-RADONC-PHYS-RES/trackrad2025
11. Wang, Y., et al.: TrackRAD 2025 challenge dataset: real-time tumor tracking for MRI-guided radiotherapy. Med. Phys. **52**(7), e17964 (2025)

An Adapted SAM2.1 Framework for Real-Time Tumor Segmentation in MRI-Guided Radiotherapy

Hung Chu(✉) and Jiapan Guo

Bernoulli Institute of Mathematics, Computer Science and Artificial Intelligence, University of Groningen, Nijenborg 9, 9747AG Groningen, The Netherlands
d.h.chu@rug.nl

Abstract. We fine-tuned the Segment Anything Model 2.1 (SAM2.1) base-plus variant [6] for real-time tumor tracking in 2D cine-MRI. The architecture was consistently applied across diverse anatomical locations and field strengths. The pre-trained SAM2.1 model, originally designed for RGB images, was adapted for single-channel grayscale MRI by averaging the weights of the vision input layer across channels. The model was primarily trained using SAM2.1's default configuration with the AdamW optimizer, base learning rate of 5e-6, vision learning rate of 3e-6, and cosine learning rate scheduler. In addition to the standard SAM2.1 loss functions (focal, Dice, mean absolute error, and cross-entropy), five domain-specific losses were implemented to improve tumor tracking: boundary, center distance, surface, temporal, and motion. A bounding box cropping strategy was used for preprocessing, with min-max normalization and SAM's default Z-score normalization applied. Data augmentation included random horizontal flips, rotations, zooms, and crops. The model was fine-tuned for 250 epochs, with the best model selected based on the highest average score on the validation set. During inference, frame intensities were clipped between the 10th and 100th percentiles of the initial frame's intensity distribution. After prediction, a 3 $\times$ 3 Gaussian filter was applied to smooth the mask boundaries. The final model achieved an average Dice similarity coefficient of 0.93 on the validation set and 0.91 on the preliminary testing set.

Keywords: Real-time tumor tracking · MRI-guided radiotherapy · Medical image segmentation · SAM2.1 · Deep learning

1 Introduction

Precise tumor targeting is crucial in radiotherapy to minimize dose to healthy tissues [4]. Effective motion management is critical for tumors affected by respiratory motion. The recent advances in MRI-guided radiotherapy (MRI-linacs) have revolutionized this field by enabling continuous, real-time visualization of tumor position during treatment through 2D cine-MRI [3]. This capability facilitates

J. P. Wachs et al. (Eds.): TrackRAD/TTC 2025, LNCS 16474, pp. 25–35, 2027.
https://doi.org/10.1007/978-3-032-35046-6_3

adaptive treatment strategies, allowing for potential dose escalation and reduced toxicity.

Despite MRI-linac advantages, accurate and robust real-time tumor tracking remains a significant challenge. Current clinical solutions, relying on conventional deformable image registration or template matching, frequently encounter difficulties with large, non-rigid tumor motion, limiting real-time adaptation effectiveness [1]. This limitation can increase treatment times and restrict the number of patients who can benefit from advanced motion management.

Artificial intelligence (AI) has advanced significantly, offering promising applications within the medical field [7]. Moreover, AI-driven approaches can potentially provide the high accuracy and robustness needed for real-time tumor segmentation. The TrackRAD2025 challenge accelerates the development and evaluation of these advanced methods [8]. The objective of the challenge is to facilitate the development of algorithms that, given the initial tumor segmentation from the first frame, can accurately segment the tumor in real-time on subsequent frames. The outcomes of TrackRAD2025 will inform the clinical adoption of more accurate tumor tracking techniques, which can lead to more efficient dose delivery and improved patient outcomes.

Given the requirements of real-time performance, high accuracy, and robustness to diverse and challenging medical imaging conditions, our approach leverages the Segment Anything Model 2.1 (SAM2.1) [6]. SAM2.1 stands out as an advanced foundation model with an architecture designed for image and video segmentation. The model includes a memory mechanism that handles common video segmentation challenges, such as object occlusion and reappearance, ensuring consistent object tracking across frames. Furthermore, its reported inference speed (with an average of 64.1 frames per second, or 15.6 ms per frame, for video object segmentation) addresses the need for rapid segmentation in cine-MRI. Therefore, we believe that SAM2.1 is an excellent candidate for handling the complex real-time tumor tracking in MRI-guided radiotherapy.

2 Methods

2.1 Data

For comprehensive details on the dataset's characteristics, please refer to the original publication by [8]. In summary, the TrackRAD2025 dataset contains 585 sagittal 2D cine-MRI sequences from six international clinical centers (Netherlands, Germany, Australia, China), capturing tumors in the thorax, abdomen, and pelvis. Images were acquired using 0.35T MRIdian and 1.5T Unity MRI-linac systems. The dataset is split into a public training set (527 cases: 477 unlabeled, 50 labeled) and a private testing set (58 labeled cases). Scans include breath holds and free breathing. Challenges include treatment interruptions in 1.5T data and image degradation during gantry movement in 0.35T data, alongside varied frame rates (up to 8 Hz) and acquisition parameters.

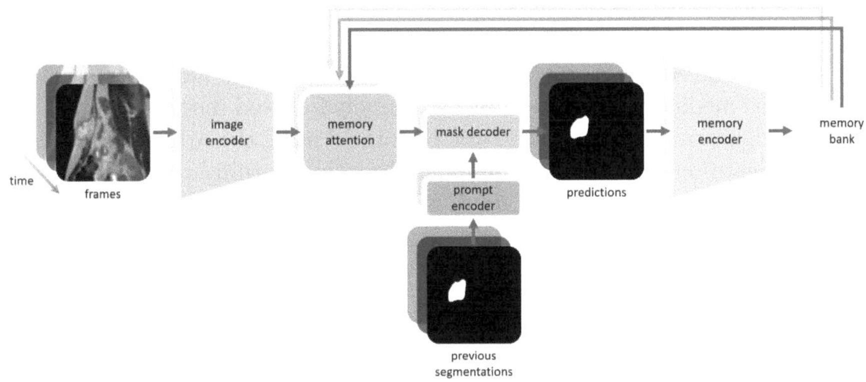

Fig. 1. This figure illustrates the SAM 2.1 architecture for this challenge.

2.2 Model

The core of the proposed methodology is the Segment Anything Model 2.1 (SAM2.1), specifically the base-plus (b+) variant [6], as illustrated in Fig. 1. This variant was chosen to achieve an optimal balance between segmentation performance and computational runtime speed. The architecture of SAM2.1 is built upon several core components:

The image encoder uses a transformer-based architecture to extract high-level features from individual cine-MRI frames. It is responsible for understanding the visual content at each timestep.

The memory mechanism processes and stores the information from the current cine-MRI frame and integrates it with the knowledge from previous frames, enabling the model to maintain consistent tumor tracking over time. This mechanism is crucial for handling temporal dependencies and common video segmentation challenges, such as small tumors and occlusions.

The prompt encoder incorporates the tumor segmentation mask of the first cine-MRI frame. The prompt encoder enables the model to adapt to user input, thereby guiding the segmentation task.

The mask decoder generates the final segmentation masks based on the encoded image features and prompt. The decoder uses a transformer network to process memory context for accurate tumor tracking across all cine-MRI frames.

As SAM2.1 was pre-trained for three-channel RGB images and the MRI data is single-channel grayscale, the model was adapted by averaging the vision input layer weights across channels. This, along with changing the mask decoder's output channels from three to one (for binary segmentation), was the only architectural modification made to the pre-trained model. The final model contains a total of 80.8M trainable parameters.

2.3 Training

The training involved fine-tuning the pre-trained SAM2.1 b+ model on the challenge's labeled medical imaging dataset. We largely followed the SAM's standard training configuration. Optimization was performed using the AdamW optimizer with a base learning rate of 5e-6 and a vision-specific learning rate of 3e-6. The cosine learning rate scheduler was used, where the end learning rate was set to one-tenth of the starting learning rate. We changed the default training configuration to run for 250 epochs, batch size of 1, and processing 16 frames per cine-MRI sequence.

Additional Loss Functions. In addition to SAM2.1's standard loss functions (focal, Dice, mean absolute error (MAE), and cross-entropy (CE)), we included five domain-specific losses to improve boundary delineation, centroid localization, and temporal consistency in cine-MRI sequences:

1. **Boundary loss** forces the model to pay extra attention to obtaining the pixels at the edge of the object correctly. This weighted binary cross-entropy (BCE) loss prioritizes pixels near the ground truth mask's boundary. Let:
   - P be the predicted probability mask.
   - T be the binary ground truth mask.
   - K be a convolution kernel of ones.
   - $\oplus$ and $\ominus$ be the morphological dilation and erosion, respectively.
   - λ be the weight multiplier.
   - N be the total number of pixels.
   - α_{boundary} be the scaling factor.

   The boundary region B of the ground truth mask is calculated as:

   $$B = (T \oplus K) \setminus (T \ominus K) \tag{1}$$

   The weight map W is defined as:

   $$W_{xy} = 1 + (\lambda - 1) \cdot B_{xy} \tag{2}$$

   The boundary-aware loss is the weighted BCE:

   $$\mathcal{L}_{\text{boundary}} = -\alpha_{\text{boundary}} \cdot \frac{1}{N} \sum_{i=1}^{N} W_i \left[T_i \log(P_i) + (1 - T_i) \log(1 - P_i)\right] \tag{3}$$

2. **Center distance loss** encourages the predicted mask to follow the object as it moves across frames, preventing it from drifting away. Moreover, this loss penalizes the Euclidean distance between the center of mass of the predicted mask and the ground truth mask. Let:
   - P be the predicted probability mask.
   - T be the binary ground truth mask.
   - c be the 2D coordinate vector.
   - α_{cd} be the scaling factor.

The center of mass for the predicted mask (C_P) and the ground truth mask (C_T) are calculated as the weighted average of pixel coordinates:

$$C_P = \frac{\sum_i P_i \cdot c_i}{\sum_i P_i}, \quad C_T = \frac{\sum_i T_i \cdot c_i}{\sum_i T_i} \tag{4}$$

The center distance loss is the L_2 norm of the difference between the centers of mass:

$$\mathcal{L}_{\text{center}} = \alpha_{\text{cd}} \cdot \|C_P - C_T\|_2 \tag{5}$$

3. **Surface loss** penalizes errors based on their distance from the correct boundary, unlike Dice or CE loss, which treat all misclassified pixels equally. Moreover, this loss uses Signed Distance Transforms (SDT) to penalize discrepancies at the object boundaries. Let:
   - P be the predicted probability mask.
   - T be the binary ground truth mask.
   - ϕ_P be the SDT of the predicted mask P.
   - ϕ_T be the SDT of the ground truth mask T.
   - N be the total number of pixels.
   - α_{surface} be the scaling factor.

   The surface loss is defined as the integral of the absolute difference between the predicted probabilities and the ground truth, weighted by the distance maps:

$$\mathcal{L}_{\text{surface}} = \alpha_{\text{surface}} \cdot \frac{1}{N} \sum_{i=1}^{N} |P_i \phi_{T,i} + (1 - P_i)\phi_{P,i}| \tag{6}$$

4. **Temporal loss** encourages smoothness between predicted masks in consecutive frames by penalizing the absolute difference. Let:
   - P_t be the predicted probability mask at the current time step t.
   - P_{t-1} be the predicted probability mask at the previous time step $t-1$.
   - N be the total number of pixels.
   - α_{temporal} be the scaling factor.

   The temporal consistency loss is the mean absolute difference between the two masks:

$$\mathcal{L}_{\text{temporal}} = \alpha_{\text{temporal}} \cdot \frac{1}{N} \sum_{i=1}^{N} |P_{t,i} - P_{t-1,i}| \tag{7}$$

5. **Motion loss** encourages the model to learn a plausible and smooth motion path. It extends beyond temporal loss by ensuring not only positional smoothness but also smooth velocity of change. Furthermore, this loss penalizes acceleration in mask changes over three consecutive frames to promote smooth motion. Let:
   - P_t, P_{t-1}, P_{t-2} be the predicted probability masks at time steps t, $t-1$, and $t-2$.

- N be the total number of pixels.
- α_{motion} be the scaling factor.

The loss is based on the L_2 norm of the second-order difference (acceleration) of the masks:

$$\mathcal{L}_{\text{motion}} = \alpha_{\text{motion}} \cdot \frac{1}{N}\|(P_t - P_{t-1}) - (P_{t-1} - P_{t-2})\|_2 \quad (8)$$

$$= \alpha_{\text{motion}} \cdot \frac{1}{N}\|P_t - 2P_{t-1} + P_{t-2}\|_2 \quad (9)$$

Data Processing. All frames underwent preprocessing to prepare them for model input; an overview of the data preprocessing is depicted in Fig. 2. Firstly, to localize the region of interest for tracking, we implemented a bounding box cropping strategy centered on the first tumor segmentation of the cine-MRI sequence. Specifically, we identify the non-zero pixels in the tumor segmentation mask of the first frame, determine the minimum spatial dimensions that encompass these pixels, and determine the center coordinate. The bounding box is cropped around the center coordinate, and the size is set to twice the minimum spatial dimensions, with a minimum size of height $\times$ width $= 128 \times 128$. The cropping window is constrained to a square aspect ratio by selecting the larger dimension, ensuring both width and height are equal.

Secondly, data augmentation techniques were used during training to enhance the model's robustness and ability to generalize across the dataset. These augmentations were applied randomly to the cropped bounding box region, each with a probability of 0.5, and consistently across all frames within the cine-MRI sequence. The techniques included random horizontal flip, random rotation up to $10°$, random zoom up to 10%, resize to 282×282 ($= 256^2 \cdot 1.10$), and crop a random region of 256×256.

Finally, intensity values were normalized to the [0, 1] pixel-value range using the min-max normalization, followed by SAM2.1's default Z-score normalization, with $\mu = 0.449$ and $\sigma = 0.226$ (i.e., the average μ and σ of the RGB channels). This standardization is a deliberate choice to ensure consistency with the pre-trained weights of the SAM2.1 model. This alignment minimizes domain shift at the input layer, which is crucial for effective fine-tuning and leveraging the general visual features learned during the extensive pre-training phase. The resulting frames with shape (frames, channels, height, width) = (16, 1, 256, 256) were used as input for the model.

During inference, two additional data processing steps were applied. First, before feeding the frames to the model, frame intensities were clipped based on the 10th and 100th percentiles of the initial frame's intensity distribution. Second, after prediction, the resulting segmentation masks were post-processed by applying a 3×3 Gaussian filter to smooth the mask boundaries.

Hyperparameter Tuning. To optimize hyperparameters and validate the model, we divided the public labeled dataset into an 80% training set and a 20% validation set, stratified by medical center. The scaling factors for the additional five losses were the hyperparameters tuned. Model checkpoints were saved

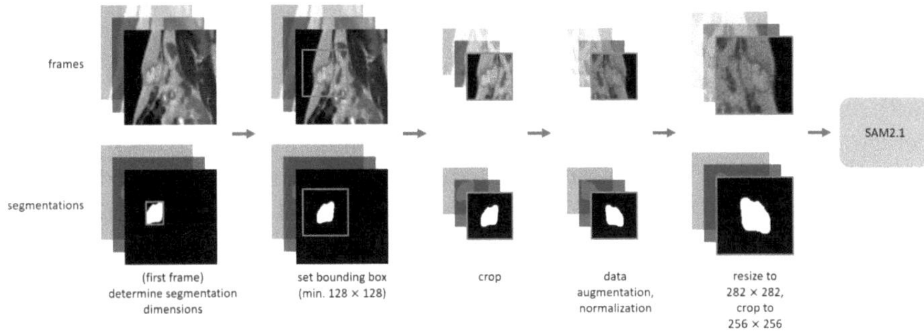

Fig. 2. Flow chart of the data preprocessing.

every 10 epochs. The best checkpoint was determined by the best average score achieved on the validation set, using the same metrics and ranking system as this challenge. The best checkpoint was trained for another 10 epochs on the full dataset (both training and validation splits) for submission to the challenge. The larger unlabeled dataset, also provided as part of the challenge, was not used in this supervised learning approach. Table 1 provides a concise overview of the model and training configuration.

Table 1. Model training configuration.

Parameter	Value/Description
Model architecture	SAM2.1 b+
Total parameters	80.8 M
In- and output channels	1
Image input size	256 × 256
Bounding box cropping	Around center of first tumor segmentation, 2x size (min. 128 × 128, square)
Epochs	250
Batch size	1
Number of frames	16
Optimizer	AdamW
Base learning rate	5e-6
Vision learning rate	3e-6
Learning rate scheduler	Cosine
Loss functions	Focal, Dice, MAE, CE, Boundary, Center distance, Surface, Temporal, Motion
Data augmentation	Random horizontal flip, rotation, zoom, and crop
Intensity normalization	SAM2.1's default Z-score normalization (μ = 0.449, $\sigma = 0.226$) and min-max normalization
Tuning hyperparameters	α_{boundary}, α_{cd}, α_{surface}, α_{temporal}, α_{motion}

2.4 Evaluation

The model's performance was assessed using four geometric metrics (Dice similarity coefficient (DSC), 95th percentile Hausdorff distance (HD95), mean average surface distance (MASD), Euclidean center distance (CD)) and one radiotherapy-specific dose metric. The runtime per frame of the model inference was considered to ensure that the model did not exceed the maximum runtime of 1 s per frame. The 95% confidence intervals ($CI_{95\%}$) were computed to quantify uncertainty in the evaluation metrics.

Software. PyTorch v2.6.0 [5] and the official SAM2.1 repository [8] were used for data preparation and modelling. MONAI v1.4.0 [2] was used for data augmentation operations. All performance metrics were computed using the challenge's evaluation code. The source code is publicly available at https://github.com/HC94/TrackRAD2025.

3 Results

3.1 Model Performance

During the tuning process, the optimal hyperparameters were determined to be $\alpha_{\text{boundary}} = 1$, $\alpha_{\text{cd}} = 1\text{e-}2$, $\alpha_{\text{surface}} = 1\text{e-}4$, $\alpha_{\text{temporal}} = 0.5$, $\alpha_{\text{motion}} = 0.3$. The model training time for 250 epochs was approximately 15 h using one NVIDIA A100 (40 GB) GPU. The performance of the resulting model on the validation and preliminary testing sets, along with their $CI_{95\%}$, is summarized in Table 2.

For the validation set, the model demonstrated a strong overall performance, with an average DSC=0.93 [$CI_{95\%}$, 0.90 – 0.95], HD95=2.54 mm [1.94 – 3.14], MASD=1.03 mm [0.79 – 1.27], CD=0.99 mm [0.74 – 1.25], and the radiotherapy-specific dose metric of 1.00 [1.00 – 1.00]. The average inference runtime was 24 ms [23 – 26] per frame, which was achieved on an NVIDIA A100 (40 GB) GPU.

In the preliminary testing phase, the model also demonstrated a strong overall performance, although slightly lower than that observed on the validation set. The average DSC was 0.91 [0.88 – 0.95], demonstrating strong volumetric overlap between the predicted segmentation and the ground truth. The boundary delineation was also precise, as indicated by low values for HD95=4.64 mm [2.51 – 6.76] and MASD=1.59 mm [0.79 – 2.38]. CD=1.77 mm [1.21 – 2.33] confirmed the model's ability to localize the tumor centroid accurately. The average value of the radiotherapy-specific dose metric was 0.97 [0.94 – 1.00].

Table 2. Quantitative performance metrics on the validation and preliminary testing set. ↑: Higher is better. ↓: Lower is better.

Metric	Validation (n =10) [$CI_{95\%}$]	Preliminary testing (n =8) [$CI_{95\%}$]
DSC (↑)	0.93	0.91
	[0.90 – 0.95]	[0.88 – 0.95]
HD95 (mm) (↓)	2.54	4.64
	[1.94 – 3.14]	[2.51 – 6.76]
MASD (mm) (↓)	1.03	1.59
	[0.79 – 1.27]	[0.79 – 2.38]
CD (mm) (↓)	0.99	1.77
	[0.74 – 1.25]	[1.21 – 2.33]
Dose (↑)	1.00	0.97
	[1.00 – 1.00]	[0.94 – 1.00]
Runtime per frame (ms) (↓)	24	–
	[23 – 26]	–

3.2 Analysis of Cine-MRI Sequences

Figure 3 presents examples of the three lowest- and highest-performing cine-MRI sequences. The frames on the left side of the figure correspond to patients with the lowest performance. The tumors in these sequences, such as those from patients A_021 (DSC=0.85) and B_012 (DSC=0.84), are notably small and exhibit low contrast with the surrounding tissue. In these instances, the model's prediction (blue) demonstrated relatively low overlap with the ground truth segmentation (orange). Despite these challenges, the model was able to track the tumor until the final frame of the sequence. For patient A_013 (DSC=0.81), the ground truth segmentation was absent from frame 87 onwards (until frame 100) while the model continued to make predictions, resulting in lower metric values.

The frames on the right side of the figure represent the best-performing sequences, characterized by a high degree of overlap between the predicted segmentations and the ground truth. These sequences achieved a high DSC ranging from 0.97 to 0.98. The model successfully tracked the tumor over all frames, which could be attributed to the larger tumor size and higher contrast of the surrounding tissue.

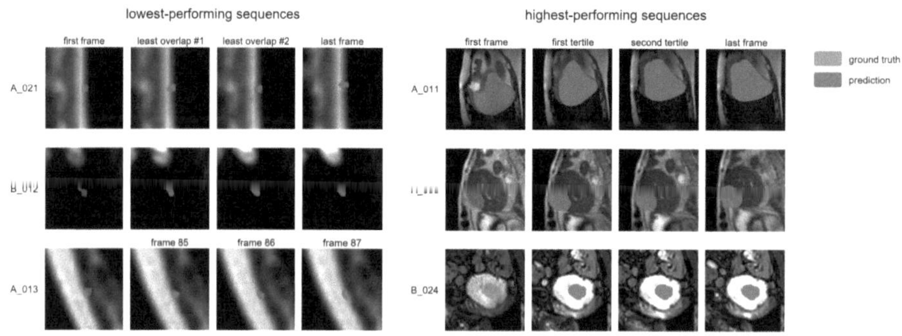

Fig. 3. Examples of the lowest- and highest-performing cine-MRI sequences. The left side of the figure shows the three lowest-performing sequences. For patients A_021 (DSC=0.85) and B_012 (DSC=0.84), frames with the least overlap between the ground truth (orange) and the model's prediction (blue) are shown. Patient A_013's (DSC=0.81) example illustrates the challenge where the ground truth segmentation is absent from frame 87 onwards. The right side of the figure shows the best-performing sequences with DSC between 0.97 and 0.98. For all sequences, the first frame only displays the ground truth segmentation and not the model's prediction, because the first frame segmentation is provided as the model input. (Color figure online)

4 Discussion

The results demonstrate that the adapted SAM2.1 b+ model is capable of performing real-time tumor tracking accurately and efficiently. The proposed model achieved a high DSC score (0.93 [0.90 – 0.95] on validation; 0.91 [0.88 – 0.95] on testing), indicating excellent volumetric overlap between the real and predicted tumor segmentations (Table 2). The model achieved good scores for HD95 (2.54 mm [1.94 – 3.14] on validation; 4.64 mm [2.51 – 6.76] on testing) and MASD (1.03 mm [0.79 – 1.27 on validation; 1.59 mm [0.79 – 2.38] on testing). These low HD95 and MASD values imply precise boundary delineation, which is essential for minimizing radiation exposure to surrounding healthy tissues and organs-at-risk. Furthermore, tumor localization was accurate, as indicated by the low Euclidean center distances (0.99 mm [0.74 – 1.25] on validation; 1.77 mm [1.21 – 2.33] on testing). Dose metrics further confirmed clinical utility, with near-optimal scores (1.00 [1.00 – 1.00] on validation; 0.97 [0.94 – 1.00] on testing), directly linking segmentation accuracy to effective radiation delivery. Real-time feasibility was ensured by an average inference time of 24 ms [23 – 26] per frame on an NVIDIA A100 (40 GB) GPU, significantly below the 125 ms requirement for 8 Hz cine-MRI. Although slight performance declines were observed on the preliminary testing set, the model maintained strong overall accuracy.

Despite the promising performance, the study identified several limitations. The model's performance was observed to degrade when confronted with cine-MRI sequences containing small tumors, those with low contrast against the background, and instances where the ground truth segmentation was absent in several frames (Fig. 3). The analysis also revealed that while the model performed well on a diverse dataset, its performance was better for larger tumors with higher contrast. Future research is suggested to focus on developing models capable of effectively handling these challenging cases, potentially by integrating image enhancement techniques or by incorporating prior knowledge of tumor dynamics.

Acknowledgement. We thank the Center for Information Technology of the University of Groningen for their support and for providing access to the Hábrók high performance computing cluster.

Author contributions. Hung Chu was responsible for the Conceptualization, Data curation, Formal analysis, Investigation, Methodology, Project administration, Software, Validation, Visualization, and Writing – original draft. Jiapan Guo was responsible for Funding acquisition, Resources, Supervision, and Writing – review & editing.

Disclosure of Interests. The authors have no competing interests to declare that are relevant to the content of this article.

References

1. Brock, K., Oldham, M., Pouliot, J., Cai, J.: TH-C-BRF-01: the promise and potential pitfalls of deformable image registration in clinical practice. Med. Phys. **41**, 553–553 (2014). https://doi.org/10.1118/1.4889611
2. Cardoso, M.J., et al.: MonAI: an open-source framework for deep learning in healthcare (2022). https://doi.org/10.48550/arXiv.2211.02701
3. Keall, P.J., et al.: Integrated MRI-guided radiotherapy – opportunities and challenges. Nat. Rev. Clin. Oncol. **19**, 458–470 (2022). https://doi.org/10.1038/s41571-022-00631-3
4. Mirestean, C.C., Buzea, C.G., Iancu, R.I., Iancu, D.P.T.: Implications of radiosensitizer and radioprotector factors in refining the dose-volume constraints and radiobiological models. IntechOpen (2021). https://doi.org/10.5772/intechopen.89829
5. Paszke, A., et al.: PyTorch: an imperative style, high-performance deep learning library. In: Advances in Neural Information Processing Systems. Curran Associates, Inc. (2019). https://doi.org/10.48550/arXiv.1912.01703
6. Ravi, N.,et al.: SAM 2: segment anything in images and videos. In: The International Conference on Learning Representations (2024)
7. Sabbar, H., Silkan, H., Abbad, K., Bellfkih, E.M., EddineIdrissi, I.C.: Overview of medical image segmentation techniques through artificial intelligence and computer vision. Int. J. Comput. Digit. Syst. **15**, 1135–1146 (2024). https://doi.org/10.12785/ijcds/160183
8. Wang, Y., et al.: TrackRAD2025 challenge dataset: real-time tumor tracking for MRI-guided radiotherapy. Med. Phys. **52** (2025). https://doi.org/10.1002/mp.17964

No Chains, Just Gains: Ensembled SAM2.1 Motion-Tracking for Cine-MRI (TrackRAD 2025)

Maximilian Nielsen and Thilo Sentker(✉)

Institute for Applied Medical Informatics, University Medical Center Hamburg-Eppendorf, Hamburg, Germany
{m.nielsen,t.sentker}@uke.de

Abstract. We propose a deep learning-based tumor tracking pipeline for cine-MRI within the TrackRAD 2025 challenge. Our method builds upon the Segment Anything Model (SAM2.1) and utilizes a ensembling temporal motion-tracking framework that leverages the provided initial tumor mask in the first frame. We fine-tuned three SAM2.1 variants (tiny, small, base+) using challenge data and ensembled their framewise logits for robust segmentation over time. Our pipeline is anatomy-agnostic and was applied consistently across all anatomical regions and field strengths. Preprocessing included z-score intensity normalization and definition of regions of interest. Post-processing involved soft-label averaging and morphological refinement. The approach achieved high temporal stability and spatial accuracy, ranking 1st in the validation phase and achieving a top-5 ranking on the final test set leaderboard. We further discuss the trade-offs between leaderboard optimization and clinical reality, specifically regarding real-time causality and out-of-plane motion detection.

Keywords: TrackRAD 2025 · SAM2 · cine-MRI · motion tracking

1 Introduction

Magnetic resonance imaging (MRI)-guided radiotherapy represents a paradigm shift in oncology, particularly through the advent of hybrid MRI-linear accelerator (MRI-linac) systems. These platforms allow for the visualization of soft-tissue contrast during treatment delivery, enabling the monitoring of intrafractional tumor motion. This capability is relevant for thoracic and abdominal tumors, where respiratory motion can cause significant displacement, necessitating larger safety margins that inadvertently irradiate healthy tissue. TrackRAD 2025 builds upon this technological leap by providing a rich, multi-institutional dataset of sagittal 2D cine-MRI sequences acquired from six international centers [1].

The challenge of tracking tumors in 2D cine-MRI is compounded by low temporal resolution, artifacts, and out-of-plane motion. Traditional registration-based methods, such as deformable image registration or template matching,

J. P. Wachs et al. (Eds.): TrackRAD/TTC 2025, LNCS 16474, pp. 36–42, 2027.
https://doi.org/10.1007/978-3-032-35046-6_4

focus on frame alignment but often struggle with large, non-rigid anatomical deformations and the drift associated with long sequences.

In this work, we propose a strictly causal tracking framework that propagates tumor masks across cine-MRI frames by leveraging the semantic consistency and motion sensitivity inherent in foundation models. Specifically, we adapt the Segment Anything Model 2.1 (SAM2.1) [2], a vision foundation model, for the specific domain of medical tumor tracking. By fine-tuning an ensemble of SAM2.1 variants and integrating a temporal consistency term, our method balances the high feature expressiveness of large-scale pretraining with the temporal stability required for clinical safety.

2 Methods

2.1 Data Description

We utilized a subset of the TrackRAD 2025 training set, consisting of 50 labeled 2D+t cine-MRI sequences. Each labeled sequence contains manual tumor annotations for all frames in the training set. The primary input to our pipeline is the raw cine-MRI frames plus the ground-truth mask of the very first frame, which serves as the initialization seed. We did not use any of the provided unlabeled data or any external datasets. For intermediate validation and hyperparameter tuning, we utilized the 8 validation cases provided by the organizers [3].

2.2 Preprocessing

During preprocessing, image intensities within each sequence were z-score normalized to reduce variability across scans. To focus the model on relevant anatomy, a spatial bounding box was computed around the initial tumor mask in the first frame. This box was centered on the tumor centroid and padded with a 100-pixel margin. The final crop size was determined dynamically: if the padded box dimensions were smaller than 256 pixels, a crop of 256×256 pixels was used; otherwise, a size of 512×512 pixels was selected. This strategy ensured that small tumors retained sufficient spatial context for boundary delineation while guaranteeing that large tumors were fully captured. Finally, all cropped inputs were resized to a standard resolution of 1024×1024 pixels.

2.3 Model Architecture and Pipeline Overview

Our tracking framework employs an ensemble of three SAM2.1 variants: *tiny*, *small*, and *base+* [2]. The *large* variant was excluded due to computational constraints. Each model processes the cine-MRI sequence independently before their outputs are fused. The system functionality is schematically illustrated in Fig. 1.

The core tracking mechanism operates on a strict frame-by-frame basis, where the prediction for the current frame informs the input for the next. First, the initial ground truth mask provided in frame $t = 0$ is encoded into sparse and dense embedding representations to initialize the tracker. For subsequent frames

$t > 0$, each model predicts the new mask position based on the image features of the current frame t and a memory bank of features accumulated from previous frames. We emphasize temporal consistency checks, penalizing predictions that deviate abruptly or unrealistically from the trajectory defined by previous high-confidence frames.

2.4 Temporal Fusion, Frame Ensembling and Post-processing

To combine the outputs of the three models, we implement a soft-voting strategy. At each time step t, the raw segmentation logits from the tiny, small, and base+ models are averaged.

Following this spatial aggregation, we apply a temporal fusion step to smooth the trajectory. The logit map at the current frame, L_t^{ensemble}, is updated using a momentum-based approach with the final logits from the previous frame, L_{t-1}^{final}:

$$L_t^{\text{final}} = (1 - \alpha) \cdot L_t^{\text{ensemble}} + \alpha \cdot L_{t-1}^{\text{final}} \tag{1}$$

The smoothing factor α adapts to the frame rate of the MRI sequence. For high-frequency acquisition (8 fps), where inter-frame motion is minimal, we use a higher $\alpha = 0.4$ to stabilize boundaries. For slow acquisition (1 fps), where significant motion can occur between frames, α is reduced to 0.1. For intermediate frame rates, α is determined via linear interpolation.

Finally, the fused logits are passed through a sigmoid activation. A morphological binary closing operation is applied to the thresholded (0.5) mask to fill small holes and smooth jagged edges, producing the final binary prediction. Crucially, this final binary mask is fed back to each of the three SAM2.1 variants as the dense mask prompt for the next time step. This ensures that the robust ensemble consensus, rather than any single model's raw output, serves as the reference for future predictions.

The respective source code can be found on GitHub.

3 Experiments and Results

3.1 Training and Fine-Tuning

We conducted baseline experiments to determine the optimal configuration before fine-tuning. The models were full fine-tuned using the labeled training subset. To prevent overfitting to the specific training anatomies, we applied heavy data augmentation, including random affine transformations, flips, and intensity shifting. The ensemble was trained for 450 epochs, which was empirically determined to offer the best trade-off between convergence and generalization; training for 1000 epochs resulted in overfitting. Optimization was performed using AdamW with a cosine decay learning rate schedule starting at 1×10^{-4}.

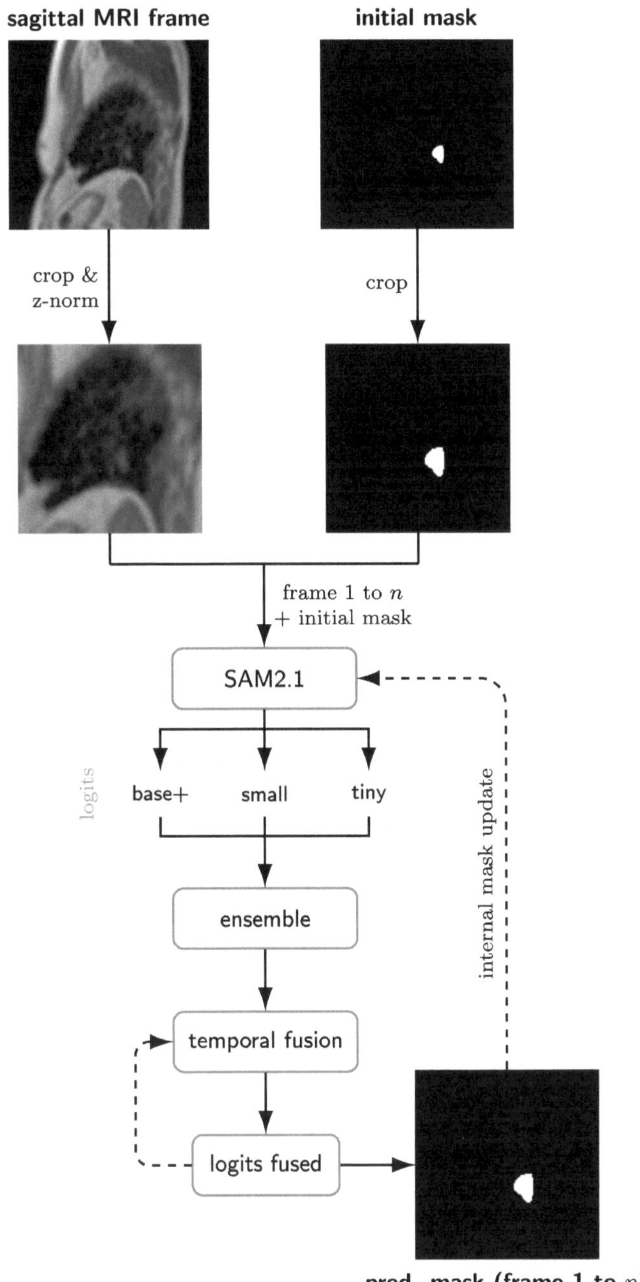

Fig. 1. Overview of the tumor tracking pipeline: starting from an initial mask on the first sagittal MRI frame, cropped and normalized inputs are processed by SAM2.1 models (tiny, small, base+), ensembled, and temporally fused to generate predicted masks for all frames.

3.2 Evaluation Strategy

Given the limited training data ($n = 50$), we omitted an internal validation split and trained on the full dataset to capture the maximal range of anatomical and motion heterogeneity. Performance verification therefore relied exclusively on the official challenge validation set ($n = 8$). As the platform imposed a strict limit of 11 submissions, standard epoch-wise monitoring was infeasible. To optimize the allocation of the available submission attempts, we prioritized an ablation-style validation of pipeline components over extensive hyperparameter sweeping. Baseline performance was established with fine-tuned models at 450 epochs. Subsequent submissions incrementally integrated the temporal fusion, multi-model ensemble, and model finetuning. This stepwise protocol isolated the contribution of each module, with consecutive submissions demonstrating consistent metric improvements (see Table 1).

Table 1. Ablation study on the TrackRAD validation set. We analyze the contribution of different components to the final performance. The baseline is a standard SAM model. Subsequent rows show the impact of adding temporal information, ensembling, and finetuning. The best performance is achieved with the fully finetuned approach.

	Components				Metrics	
Method	Vanilla SAM	Temporal Fusion	Ensemble	Fine-tuning	DSC	Mean Pos.
Baseline	✓	×	×	×	0.904	47.8
+ Temporal	✓	✓	×	×	0.914	23.6
+ Ensemble	✓	✓	✓	×	0.918	13.4
+ Finetune	✓	✓	✓	✓	**0.924**	**1.4**

3.3 Quantitative Results

Our method was evaluated on two distinct sets: the validation set (during the development phase) and the held-out test set (final leaderboard). Table 2 summarizes the performance across both sets.

On the validation set, the SAM2.1 ensemble demonstrated robust tracking capabilities, achieving a mean leaderboard position of 1.4. The approach ranked first in both Average Center Distance (1.43 mm) and Average Surface Distance (1.31 mm), and secured the second rank for the Dice Similarity Coefficient (DSC) with a score of 0.9238.

On the test set, the method achieved a mean leaderboard ranking of 6.5. While the DSC remained competitive at 0.8801 (Rank 3), distance-based metrics exhibited a notable increase; specifically, the Average Center Distance rose to 2.10 mm and the 95% Surface Distance to 5.64 mm. Analysis of the individual test cases reveals that this performance drop was not driven by a systemic failure

Table 2. Comparison of results on the TrackRAD 2025 validation set versus the final test set. While the method achieved top-tier performance on the validation set, a generalization gap is observed in the final testing phase.

	Validation Set		Test Set	
Metric	Value	Rank	Value	Rank
Dice Similarity Coefficient	0.9238	2	0.8801	3
Avg. Center Distance [mm]	1.4312	1	2.1031	5
Relative D98 Dose	0.9869	2	0.9321	5
95% Surface Distance [mm]	3.8686	1	5.6407	7
Avg. Surface Distance [mm]	1.3125	1	2.2416	5
Runtime [s]	–	–	0.5155	14
Mean Leaderboard Position	–	**1.4**	–	**6.5**

to handle unseen motion patterns or artifacts, but rather by three singular failure cases.

In these specific instances, the tumor was temporarily located at the periphery of the imaging plane and was only minimally visible. The model incorrectly predicted these slices as containing no tumor (empty plane). Under the challenge evaluation metric, such false negatives are penalized with default maximum error values. Consequently, these three outliers disproportionately skewed the aggregate distance metrics, masking otherwise stable tracking performance across the majority of the test cohort.

4 Discussion

The results demonstrate that employing pretrained vision foundation models like SAM2.1 provides a robust baseline for medical object tracking. However, the discrepancy between our validation and test results highlights the complexity of the TrackRAD challenge. Beyond pure metric performance, we identify two critical areas where the design of tracking algorithms must balance leaderboard optimization against clinical reality.

A defining feature of our pipeline is the use of a foundation model ensemble strictly within an online, frame-by-frame inference loop, a necessary adaptation of the standard SAM2.1 implementation which expects complete video inputs. While this approach maximizes segmentation robustness, it resulted in a lower runtime ranking (0.5155 s per frame, Rank 14). This latency is primarily driven by the computational cost of inferencing multiple model instances in parallel, combined with the overhead of consensus voting and post-processing steps. In a clinical MRI-linac scenario, the system must process incoming images instantaneously to gate the beam. Consequently, our results highlight a trade-off: while the ensemble ensures high precision, future deployment would require distilling this performance into a single, lighter model to meet the strict latency constraints of clinical beam-gating systems.

A major challenge in cine-MRI is out-of-plane motion, where the tumor moves entirely out of the 2D sagittal slice. In these cases, the ground truth mask is empty. Correctly identifying this state is vital for safety (beam-off). However, we observed that the challenge metrics are highly volatile in these scenarios. If the algorithm predicts empty but there is a tiny remnant of tumor visible (or vice versa), metrics default to maximum penalty value. Conversely, if the algorithm simply copies the mask from the previous frame, it often secures a more optimal metric-score because the tumor location rarely changes instantly. This creates an unreasonable incentive: algorithms are rewarded on the leaderboard for propagating masks even when the tumor might be gone, whereas a clinically safe algorithm that aggressively shuts off (predicts empty) risks a metric penalty. We suggest future challenges incorporate a specific beam-gating accuracy metric to reward the correct identification of empty frames, distinct from geometric overlap.

4.1 Conclusion

We presented a SAM2.1-based ensemble for real-time tumor tracking. Our method achieved top-tier performance on the validation set and robust results on the test set. Future work will focus on closing the generalization gap via domain adaptation and optimizing the inference loop for lower latency, ensuring that high-accuracy deep learning models can be safely integrated into real-time radiotherapy workflows.

Author contributions.
Conceptualization: MN, TS
Methodology: MN, TS
Software: MN, TS
Validation: MN, TS
Formal Analysis: MN, TS
Investigation: MN, TS
Writing – Original Draft: MN, TS
Writing – Review & Editing: MN, TS
Supervision: MN, TS
Funding Acquisition: MN, TS

References

1. Keall, P.J., et al.: Integrated MRI-guided radiotherapy–opportunities and challenges. Nat. Rev. Clin. Oncol. **19**(7), 458–470 (2022)
2. Ravi, N., et al.: SAM 2: segment anything in images and videos. arXiv preprint: arXiv:2408.00714 (2024)
3. Wang, Y., et al.: TrackRAD2025 challenge dataset: real-time tumor tracking for MRI-guided radiotherapy. Med. Phys. **52**(7) (2025)
4. Zhu, J., Hamdi, A., Qi, Y., Jin, Y., Wu, J.: Medical SAM 2: segment medical images as video via segment anything model 2. arXiv preprint: arXiv:2408.00874 (2024)

Fine-Tuning Segment Anything for Real-Time Tumor Tracking in Cine-MRI

Valentin Boussot(✉), Cédric Hémon, Jean-Claude Nunes, and Jean-Louis Dillenseger

Univ Rennes 1, CLCC Eugène Marquis, INSERM, LTSI - UMR 1099, 35000 Rennes, France
boussot.v@gmail.com
https://ltsi.univ-rennes.fr/

Abstract. In this work, we address the TrackRAD2025 challenge of real-time tumor tracking in cine-MRI sequences of the thoracic and abdominal regions under strong data scarcity constraints. Two complementary strategies were explored: (i) unsupervised registration with the IMPACT similarity metric and (ii) foundation model–based segmentation leveraging SAM 2.1 and its recent variants through prompt-based interaction. Due to the one-second runtime constraint, the SAM-based method was ultimately selected. The final configuration used SAM2.1b+ with mask-based prompts from the first annotated slice, fine-tuned solely on the small labeled subset from TrackRAD2025. Training was configured to minimize overfitting, using 1024×1024 patches (batch size 1), standard augmentations, and a balanced Dice + IoU loss. A low uniform learning rate (1×10^{-5}) was applied to all modules (prompt encoder, decoder, Hiera backbone) to preserve generalization while adapting to annotator-specific styles. Training lasted 300 epochs (12h on RTX A6000, 48GB). The same inference strategy was consistently applied across all anatomical sites and MRI field strengths. Test-time augmentation was considered but ultimately discarded due to negligible performance gains. The final model was selected based on the highest Dice Similarity Coefficient achieved on the validation set after fine-tuning. On the hidden test set, the model reached a Dice score of 0.8794, ranking 6th overall in the TrackRAD2025 challenge. These results highlight the strong potential of foundation models for accurate and real-time tumor tracking in MRI-guided radiotherapy.

1 Introduction

Medical image segmentation and registration play a crucial role in numerous clinical workflows, enabling accurate delineation of anatomical structures and pathological regions for diagnosis, treatment planning, and follow-up [3,8]. In the context of the TrackRAD2025 challenge [9], the task focuses on real-time tumor tracking in 2D cine-MRI sequences of the thoracic and abdominal regions. Only

J. P. Wachs et al. (Eds.): TrackRAD/TTC 2025, LNCS 16474, pp. 43–51, 2027.
https://doi.org/10.1007/978-3-032-35046-6_5

the first frame of each sequence is annotated, and the objective is to automatically segment the tumor in all subsequent frames under fast respiratory motion and strict runtime constraints (one second per sequence). This setting reflects the clinical requirement of online motion monitoring during MRI-guided radiotherapy.

A key constraint in this challenge is the scarcity of annotated training data, which limits the applicability of conventional supervised deep learning methods that typically rely on large-scale, fully annotated datasets to reach state-of-the-art performance [5].

Given these constraints, we adopted a dual methodological strategy developed using KonfAI [1]:

- An unsupervised registration approach based on IMPACT [2], which leverages deformable image registration to propagate the initial mask across subsequent frames in the temporal sequences without requiring additional manual annotations.
- The use of foundation segmentation models, such as SAM [4] (Segment Anything Model) and MedSAM [7], which are trained on large and diverse datasets and can generalize to novel imaging modalities and anatomical sites.

The unsupervised nature of the registration approach eliminates the need for model training and parameter tuning on the challenge dataset, making it inherently robust to data scarcity. In parallel, the use of foundation models [5] provides a strong prior for anatomical segmentation [6], with the possibility of refining their performance through fine-tuning on the small annotated subset available.

This dual approach enables a direct comparison between the spatial consistency achieved through registration and the flexibility of prompted segmentation models, supporting accurate and generalizable tumor tracking in cine-MRI under limited data conditions.

2 Methods

2.1 Data

We used only the manually annotated subset of the TrackRAD2025 dataset [9]. The dataset is a multi-center collection of sagittal 2D cine-MRI sequences acquired during MRI-guided radiotherapy on two MRI-linac systems (0.35 T ViewRay MRIdian and 1.5 T Elekta Unity) across six centers. It covers thoracic (32%), abdominal (41%), and pelvic (27%) tumors. Each sequence consists of 20 to over 20000 temporal frames, sampled at 1–8 Hz depending on the vendor and acquisition protocol, capturing one or several respiratory cycles. Among the full dataset of 585 patients, 108 cases are fully annotated. In this work, we relied exclusively on the 50 publicly released annotated training cases. No unlabeled or external data were used.

2.2 Model

Unsupervised Registration with IMPACT. IMPACT is a similarity metric specifically designed for multimodal medical image registration. It leverages high-level anatomical features extracted from large, pretrained segmentation models to guide the registration process. By integrating these semantic representations, IMPACT mitigates the limitations of traditional intensity-based similarity measures, which are often sensitive to noise, artifacts, and modality-specific intensity variations.

IMPACT was integrated into the Elastix registration framework, enabling deformable image registration between frames in a cine-MRI sequence. This approach aimed to propagate the initial mask provided for the first slice to all subsequent frames via spatial transformations estimated through registration.

While theoretically well-suited to the problem, the method faced practical constraints: the challenge imposes a one-second prediction time limit per case, which required a drastic reduction in the number of optimization iterations. Despite parameter tuning, this time constraint significantly degraded the achievable registration accuracy, preventing the full exploitation of IMPACT's potential. Accordingly, we focus on the second approach, which aligns better with the challenge's runtime constraints.

Tracking with SAM. For the use of segmentation foundation models, we tested many of these models that have been validated on the available annotated dataset. The SAM, MedSAM2 models and other variants were tested on the validation dataset. We then tested several prompting techniques (point sample, box, mask of the first slice) and kept the last method using the first slice. The use of test-time augmentation was also tested but did not yield any significant improvement. The same method was used for all anatomical locations and different MRI field strengths. The average inference time per cine MRI frame was approximately 10 ms on our hardware.

The model SAM2.1 b+ was then fine-tuned as explained in the following section.

2.3 Training

During initial experiments using SAM for inference, we observed that the predictions were generally accurate. However, manual annotations consistently overestimated the segmented tumor volumes compared to SAM outputs. To account for this annotator bias, we fine-tuned the model on the labeled subset, enabling it to learn this discrepancy and align its predictions with the provided ground truth masks.

Fine-tuning was performed following the specific training requirements of the SAM architecture. Input patches of size 1024×1024 were extracted from the cine MRI sequences. Standard data augmentation techniques were applied, including RandomHorizontalFlip, RandomAffine, ColorJitter, and RandomGrayscale, to improve generalization and robustness. The model was trained with a batch size of 1 and supervised using a composite loss combining Dice loss (weight=1) and IoU loss (weight=1). Optimization was performed using the AdamW optimizer. Sequences of 8 consecutive frames (number of frames = 8) were provided as input.

The training procedure employed binary masks as prompts, with a learning rate of 0.0005 for the prompt network, the decoder, and the Hiera based encoder. This relatively low learning rate was selected to preserve the pretrained capabilities of SAM while enabling it to adapt to the mask-prompt bias present in the training data.

The model was trained for 300 epochs, and the network from the final epoch was selected as the deployed model for subsequent evaluations. Training required approximately 12 h in total on an NVIDIA RTX A6000 GPU (48 GB).

2.4 Evaluation

To assess the quality of tumor tracking in the TrackRAD2025 challenge, we employed the full set of evaluation metrics defined by the challenge organizers. These metrics aim to quantify both segmentation fidelity and the geometric accuracy of temporal tracking. They include:

- **Dice Similarity Coefficient (DSC)**: Measures the spatial overlap between the predicted and reference masks, defined as twice the intersection divided by the sum of their volumes:

$$\text{DSC} = \frac{2|A \cap B|}{|A| + |B|}$$

  A higher DSC (maximum value of 1) indicates stronger agreement. This metric is widely used in medical image segmentation.
- **Hausdorff Distance (HD)** and **Average Surface Distance (ASD)**: These metrics evaluate the distance between the surfaces of the predicted and reference masks. HD measures the largest surface-to-surface distance, while ASD reports the average distance, providing a more stable indicator of contour accuracy.
- **Center of Mass Distance (CD)**: The Euclidean distance between the centroids of the predicted and reference segmentations. This captures the spatial consistency of tracking over time.
- **Inference Speed**: Given that real-time performance is a critical requirement in this challenge, the inference speed of the method is recorded. The competition imposes a maximum prediction time per case (approximately one second), making this a decisive performance criterion.
- **Estimated Radiation Dose Delivery Accuracy**: Although less common in traditional segmentation benchmarks, this metric quantifies the clinical impact of segmentation on the ability to deliver the prescribed radiotherapy dose accurately. It is included in the challenge to reflect the ultimate clinical goal of real-time treatment adaptation.

This combination of classical segmentation metrics (DSC, HD, ASD), temporal tracking measures (CD, inference speed), and clinical impact assessment (dose delivery accuracy) provides a comprehensive framework for evaluating real-time tumor tracking methods.

3 Results

We evaluated the proposed method on the TrackRAD2025 validation set using the metrics described in Sect. 2.4, excluding dose-related metrics.

To assess the potential of registration-based tumor tracking, we evaluated our IMPACT semantic similarity metric within the Elastix framework. The registration is performed between the first frame and the current frame for which the mask is propagated. A two-resolution B-spline transformation is used, with a control-point spacing of 12 mm. At each iteration, 500 voxels are randomly sampled to evaluate the similarity metric. The optimization runs for 200 iterations per resolution level. IMPACT is configured with the SAM-2.1-Small model, using two feature layers in Jacobian mode. As shown in Table 1, IMPACT noticeably improves mask propagation accuracy compared to a baseline without registration, achieving a DSC of 0.88 and reducing the Hausdorff distance by almost 50%. However, the optimization runtime currently exceeds the real-time requirement of the TrackRAD2025 challenge (one second per cine-MRI sequence), making this approach incompatible with the official constraints. For this reason, we further focused on the fine-tuned SAM-based segmentation strategy for our final submission.

Table 1. Registration-based tumor tracking performance with unrestricted runtime (not compatible with the 1-second real-time constraint).

Method	DSC ↑	HD [mm] ↓	ASD [mm] ↓	CD [mm] ↓
Baseline	0.770	8.27	3.88	6.42
IMPACT	**0.8821**	**4.4314**	**1.7868**	**2.3126**

We then compared different SAM-based configurations and prompt strategies to identify the optimal setup for the challenge constraints. Table 2 reports the performance of different foundation model configurations. The best-performing baseline was obtained with the SAM 2.1 l configuration, which achieved a DSC of 0.916, a Hausdorff Distance of 3.26 mm, an Average Surface Distance of 1.20 mm, and a Center of Mass Distance of 1.34 mm. MedSAM-based variants performed worse across all metrics, particularly in terms of distance measures. Although pretrained SAM models already yielded strong segmentation results, a systematic overestimation of tumor volume was observed in the manual annotations compared to the model predictions. This discrepancy motivated the use of fine-tuning to adapt the model to the annotator style and improve alignment with the provided ground truth. We also evaluated an ensemble prompt strategy on the SAM2.1b+ model, combining dilated and eroded versions of the initial mask to enhance robustness. However, this approach did not outperform the best model and slightly degraded performance in some metrics.

Table 2. Comparison of different prompted foundation models for segmentation on the validation set. Best values per metric are in bold.

Model	DSC ↑	HD [mm] ↓	ASD [mm] ↓	CD [mm] ↓
Baseline	0.770	8.27	3.88	6.42
SAM 2.1 t	0.911	3.45	1.27	1.51
SAM 2.1 b+	0.915	3.41	1.29	1.46
SAM 2.1 l	**0.916**	**3.26**	**1.20**	**1.34**
MedSAM2	0.869	19.76	17.01	17.28
MedSAM2 liver	0.842	29.62	27.32	27.51
Ensemble prompt	0.908	3.51	1.29	1.39

We then investigated the effect of fine-tuning SAM2.1l to better match the annotator style. As shown in Table 3, the evaluation on the training subset showed consistent improvements across all metrics, with DSC increasing from 0.916 to 0.929 and HD decreasing from 3.26mm to 2.78mm. These gains, while expected on the training set, indicate that the model successfully adapted to the annotation style without signs of overfitting.

Table 3. Performance before and after fine-tuning on the labeled subset. Best values per metric are in bold.

Model	DSC ↑	HD [mm] ↓	ASD [mm] ↓	CD [mm] ↓
SAM 2.1 b+	0.915	3.41	1.29	1.46
Fine-tuned SAM 2.1 b+	**0.929**	**2.78**	**1.00**	**1.16**

3.1 Preliminary Test Set Evaluation

To assess the generalization ability of the fine-tuned model, we further evaluated both versions (with and without fine-tuning) on the preliminary unseen test set provided by the organizers. As shown in Table 4, fine-tuning consistently improved all metrics, including DSC, center of mass accuracy, and shape consistency, confirming that the model adapted well to the annotator bias without overfitting.

Table 4. Preliminary test set evaluation. Fine-tuning significantly improved performance across all metrics.

Rank	Model	DSC ↑	CD [mm] ↓	Rel. D98 ↑	SD95 [mm] ↓	SDavg [mm] ↓
3rd	SAM 2.1 b+ (fine-tuned)	**0.9152**	**1.4912**	**0.9803**	4.2141	1.5008
5th	SAM 2.1 b+ (no fine-tune)	0.9039	1.8864	0.9312	4.9406	1.7000

Table 5. Final performance on the hidden TrackRAD2025 test set. Rankings per metric are in parentheses.

Rank	Team	DSC ↑	CD [mm] ↓	Rel. D98 ↑	SD95 [mm] ↓	SDavg [mm] ↓
1st	Track'n'Treat	**0.8909 (1)**	**1.4733 (1)**	0.9361 (4)	**4.2171 (1)**	**1.6642 (1)**
2nd	Hkini_Team	0.8860 (2)	1.4858 (2)	**0.9628 (1)**	4.4969 (2)	1.8565 (2)
3rd	felixknispelrwth	0.8764 (5)	1.6576 (3)	0.9250 (7)	4.5409 (3)	1.9174 (3)
4th	CIT	0.8712 (6)	1.9564 (4)	0.9392 (2)	5.2583 (4)	2.1903 (4)
5th	Reg'n'Track	0.8801 (3)	2.1031 (5)	0.9321 (5)	5.6407 (7)	2.2416 (5)
6th	BreizhTrack (ours)	0.8794 (4)	2.3192 (7)	0.9363 (3)	5.6298 (6)	2.6091 (8)
14th	lWM	0.8090 (14)	5.2809 (12)	0.7015 (14)	10.5484 (12)	4.8792 (12)

3.2 Official Challenge Results

Our final submission ranked 6th overall on the TrackRAD2025 leaderboard (Table 5). The top teams exhibited very similar performance, with differences of only 0.01–0.02 in Dice and small variations in CD and SD metrics, illustrating the highly competitive nature of the challenge.

4 Discussion

Our approach ranked among the best-performing submissions in the TrackRAD2025 challenge, showing that foundation models can be effectively adapted to real-time tumor tracking in cine-MRI despite limited annotated data. The narrow performance gap between the top teams highlights the competitiveness of this benchmark.

Dice scores above 0.91 on both the training and preliminary test sets indicated good generalization during development. On the final hidden test set, the Dice dropped to 0.8794, revealing a distribution shift between the development data and the evaluation cohort. Ranking differences across both stages suggest that performance on a small publicly labeled subset does not fully anticipate robustness to variations in tumor appearance, motion patterns, and acquisition protocols.

In addition to segmentation-based tracking, we evaluated a registration strategy using the IMPACT metric. By leveraging high-level anatomical features from pretrained segmentation networks, IMPACT effectively propagated the initial mask and achieved improved performance over a no-registration baseline on the validation data. Although slightly less accurate on average, the registration proved far more reliable and clinically reassuring, maintaining anatomically consistent results even under challenging motion. In contrast, segmentation-based tracking may occasionally exhibit unpredictable failures on difficult frames, leading to local inconsistencies. However, its optimization time exceeds the one-second real-time requirement of TrackRAD2025, which precludes its use as a primary solution under the challenge constraints.

Finally, we observed that fine-tuning on a small number of annotated cases improved performance on unseen patients. However, it remains unclear whether this improvement reflects a genuine gain in segmentation accuracy or rather an adaptation of the model to specific annotation styles. Overall, these results confirm that segmentation-based strategies currently offer the best trade-off between spatial accuracy and computational efficiency for this task, particularly when enhanced through targeted fine-tuning.

Acknowledgment. The work presented in this article was supported by the Brittany Region through its Allocations de Recherche Doctorale framework and by the French National Research Agency as part of the VATSop project (ANR-20-CE19-0015). Additionally, it was supported by a PhD scholarship Grant from Elekta AB (C.Hémon). The authors have no relevant financial or non-financial interests to disclose. While preparing this work, the authors used ChatGPT to enhance the writing structure and refine grammar. After using these tools, the authors reviewed and edited the content as needed and took full responsibility for the publication's content.

Author contributions. Conceptualization: V. Boussot, C. Hémon. Methodology: V. Boussot, C. Hémon. Software and experiments: V. Boussot. Supervision: J.-L. Dillenseger, J.-C. Nunes. Writing – original draft: V. Boussot, C. Hémon. Writing – review and editing: all authors.

Code availability. The inference code used for our TrackRAD2025 submission is publicly available at: https://github.com/vboussot/Trackrad2025. We also release the fine-tuned weights of the SAM 2.1 b+ model, trained on the annotated subset of the TrackRAD2025 dataset, at: https://huggingface.co/VBoussot/Trackrad2025. These resources allow full reproduction of our inference pipeline and challenge results.

References

1. Boussot, V., Dillenseger, J.L.: KonfAI: a modular and fully configurable framework for deep learning in medical imaging. arXiv preprint: arXiv:2508.09823 (2025)
2. Boussot, V., et al.: Impact: a generic semantic loss for multimodal medical image registration. arXiv preprint: arXiv:2503.24121 (2025)
3. Chen, X., et al.: Recent advances and clinical applications of deep learning in medical image analysis. Med. Image Anal. **79**, 102444 (2022)
4. Kirillov, A., et al.: Segment anything. In: Proceedings of the IEEE/CVF International Conference on Computer Vision, pp. 4015–4026 (2023)
5. Kolides, A., et al.: Artificial intelligence foundation and pre-trained models: fundamentals, applications, opportunities, and social impacts. Simul. Model. Pract. Theory **126** (2023)

6. Lee, H.H., et al.: Foundation models for biomedical image segmentation: a survey. arXiv preprint: arXiv:2401.07654 (2024)
7. Ma, J., He, Y., Li, F., Han, L., You, C., Wang, B.: Segment anything in medical images. Nat. Commun. **15**, 654 (2024)
8. Viergever, M.A., Maintz, J.B.A., Klein, S., Murphy, K., Staring, M., Pluim, J.P.W.: A survey of medical image registration – under review. Med. Image Anal. **33**, 140–144 (2016)
9. Wang, Y., et al.: TrackRAD 2025 challenge dataset: real-time tumor tracking for MRI-guided radiotherapy. Med. Phys. **52**(7), e17964 (2025)

Cascaded U-Net for Real-Time Deformable Registration in MRI-Guided Tumor Tracking

Jing Ni[1], Hongcheng Yang[2], Yanfei Liu[3], Xuewen Hou[2], and Haikun Qi[1](✉)

[1] School of Biomedical Engineering, ShanghaiTech University, Shanghai, China
[2] Shanghai United Imaging Healthcare Co., Ltd., Shanghai, 201815, China
[3] Shenzhen United Imaging Healthcare Co., Ltd., Shenzhen 518000, China

Abstract. Tumor tracking is a critical task in MRI-guided radiotherapy (MRIgRT), where accurate alignment of 2D cine-MRI frames is essential to account for tumor mo-tion during treatment. This study proposes a deep learning-based approach for re-al-time tumor tracking using a cascaded four-iteration VoxelMorph network, termed C-VMorph. The model is designed to progressively refine displacement vector fields (DVFs) to track tumor motion by aligning moving 2D cine-MRI frames with fixed target images. It leverages a cascaded U-Net architecture with ROI-guided supervision to focus on clinically relevant regions. The model was trained on both unlabeled and la-beled cine-MRI frames from the TrackRAD2025 challenge dataset. The loss function incorporates Mean Squared Error (MSE) for image similarity and a bending energy penalty for DVF regularization. Training was conducted using the Adam optimizer with an initial learning rate of 1e-4, with learning rate decay implemented using the step learning rate (StepLR) scheduler every 100 epochs. Data preprocessing involved center cropping, intensity normalization, and mask dilation, while post-processing applied morphological opening and closing to re-fine the output segmentation. The model was evaluated using geometric metrics such as the Dice Similarity Coefficient (DSC), surface distance, and Euclidean center distance, as well as a radiotherapy-specific dose metric. The results demonstrate that the C-VMorph is effective for real-time tumor tracking, showing strong potential for clinical applications in MRI-guided radiotherapy. The code is publicly available at https://github.com/Misswhale777/C_Morph.

Keywords: Radiation Therapy · Tracking · Deformable registration · TrackRAD2025 challenge

1 Introduction

Magnetic resonance imaging-guided radiotherapy (MRIgRT) with integrated MRI-linear accelerator (MRI-linac) systems enables continuous, high-contrast visualization of anatomy during irradiation, facilitating intra-fraction motion

J. P. Wachs et al. (Eds.): TrackRAD/TTC 2025, LNCS 16474, pp. 52–60, 2027.
https://doi.org/10.1007/978-3-032-35046-6_6

management in sites affected by respiration and other physiological motion [1–3]. Two-dimensional cine-MRI acquired at fixed planes or interleaved orthogonal 2D planes allows the treatment beam to respond to the current tumor position, either through beam gating or via multileaf collimator (MLC) tracking [4–6]. Both strategies require accurate, per-frame localization at clinically feasible frame rates, even when image contrast varies and the anatomy exhibits substantial non-rigid deformation.

Several target tracking strategies using cine-MRI have been explored. Early approaches employed rigid template matching or feature-based tracking for their simplicity and speed, but rigid templates failed to handle rotation or non-rigid motion and were prone to drift when image intensity or appearance changed across frames [7–9]. To account for non-rigid motion more effectively, traditional deformable image registration (DIR) was proposed. Traditional DIR computes the deformation between a reference and the current frame and then propagates the reference segmentation to the new frame, thus capturing complex motion [10]. However, the iterative optimization and multi-scale schemes inherent to these methods make real-time application challenging, especially in low-contrast cine-MRI.

With the advent of artificial intelligence, deep learning has emerged as a powerful alternative to these conventional strategies. Auto-segmentation and deformable registration can both be formulated within learning-based frameworks, amortizing computational cost during training and enabling fast inference at test time [11,12]. Blöcker et al. employed the SAM2 auto-segmentation model, which, once trained, demonstrated the capability of producing high-quality segmentation masks when applied to real-time cine MRI [13]. Lombardo et al. evaluated a hybrid Transformer-ConvNet model for DIR (TransMorph), featuring enhanced receptive fields and long-range dependencies and employing varied training strategies, reporting higher accuracy and faster speeds in 2D tumor tracking compared to traditional DIR [14]. In this line of work, a unified Transformer and super-resolution network (UTSRmorph) was recently proposed for 3D brain MRI, where it outperformed TransMorph by more effectively preserving fine spatial details and modeling long-range dependencies. These results suggest that UTSRmorph holds promise for adaptation to real-time tumor tracking [15].

Building on prior work, we evaluate and compare two deep learning approaches for real-time 2D tumor tracking. As a baseline, we adapt UTSR-Morph into a 2D variant for comparison. Considering that transformer-based models such as SAM generally require large number of parameters, we also explore a lightweight, purely convolutional neural network (CNN) alternative. Inspired by the success of VoxelMorph [16], we design a cascaded four-iteration architecture by applying the same module recursively for progressive refinement, which balances computational efficiency with tracking accuracy. All experiments are conducted within the TrackRAD2025 framework, which compiles cine-MRI datasets from multiple MRI-linac centers and provides a standardized platform for benchmarking real-time tracking methods.

2 Materials and Methods

2.1 Data

The dataset utilized in this study is derived from the TrackRAD2025 challenge. It comprises dynamic MRI data from 477 patients without manual labels (over 2.8 million sagittal 2D frames) and 108 patients with expert annotations (more than 10,000 labeled sagittal 2D frames, including approximately 8,000 with multi-observer annotations). The dataset consisted of dynamic MR acquisitions from three anatomical sites: thoracic (32%), abdominal (41%), and pelvic (27%), with each site contributing data from different patients.

The unlabeled cohort includes 253 cases acquired at 0.35 T (ViewRay MRIdian) and 224 cases at 1.5 T (Elekta Unity), with disease-site distribution of approximately 15% abdominal nodes or kidney, 25% liver, 30% lung, 10% pancreas, 10% prostate, 5% gynecological, and 5% rectal cancers. The labeled cohort includes 52 cases at 0.35 T and 56 cases at 1.5 T, distributed as 15% abdominal nodes or kidney, 20% liver, 30% lung, 15% pancreas, and 10% prostate.

Annotations included gross tumor volumes (GTVs) or, when tumor visibility on cine-MRI was inadequate, clinically chosen surrogate regions of interest (ROIs), such as the entire liver in place of a low-contrast lesion. To ensure steady-state imaging, the first five frames (0.35 T) or three frames (1.5 T) of each time series were discarded. For the labeled dataset, if the first frame still did not contain the tracking target (e.g., due to out-of-plane motion), we further removed consecutive frames until the target was present. Further details of the dataset are available in the official description published by the challenge organizers [17].

2.2 Pre-processing

All images provided by the challenge organizers were resampled to an in-plane resolution of 1×1 mm to ensure spatial consistency across patients. Subsequently, three additional preprocessing steps were applied prior to registration. First, the images were center-cropped to 256×256 pixels, with the cropping performed around the center of each image. The chosen size was determined through statistical analysis of the label data to ensure sufficient coverage of the majority of target regions within the dataset. Second, intensity values were normalized to the range [0, 1] to reduce inter-scan variation. Finally, the ROI mask was dilated by 5 pixels (approximately 5 mm in-plane at 1 mm resolution) to provide a margin against small misalignments and ensure full coverage of the target region.

2.3 Network Architecture

As a baseline, we adapted the 3D UTSRMorph transformer-based architecture for 2D tumor tracking [15]. In this adaptation, all 3D convolutional and attention operations were replaced with their 2D counterparts, and the super-resolution modules were reconfigured to operate in the 2D spatial domain. The encoder incorporates fusion attention blocks, in which ConvNet-based channel attention modules are embedded within multi-head self-attention layers, enabling the model to capture both local spatial features and long-range dependencies. The decoder employs successive 2D up-sampling and convolutional layers to generate displacement vector fields (DVFs), which describe the non-rigid transformations required to align each image pair. The network operates on sagittal cine-MRI frame pairs. Specifically, the first frame of a sequence is designated as the moving image, while each subsequent frame serves as the fixed image. For each pair, the model estimates DVFs that deforms the moving image toward the fixed image, and the same transformation is applied to the moving-frame mask to obtain the propagated segmentation.

For comparison with the transformer-based baseline, we implemented a lightweight CNN-based C-VMorph network, as illustrated in Fig. 1. A four-iteration cascade was adopted to balance computational efficiency with frame-to-frame alignment accuracy, which is essential for reliable real-time tumor tracking. Each iteration consists of a U-Net-like encoder-decoder module with skip connections. For each iteration beyond the first, the input to the module is formed by concatenating the previously warped moving image with the fixed image, and the module refines the DVF estimated in the previous stage. In the encoder, strided 2D convolutions with Leaky ReLU activations progressively reduce spatial resolution, allowing deeper layers to capture coarser yet contextually informative representations. In the decoder, upsampling layers are interleaved with convolutions and skip connections, propagating fine-grained encoder features to guide DVF generation at higher spatial resolutions. At each stage, a spatial transformer network (STN) applies the predicted DVF to warp the moving image. The cascade produces one DVF per iteration, and incremental fields are accumulated across iterations to form a cumulative DVF. To further emphasize clinically relevant regions, we incorporated an ROI-guided mechanism: when an ROI mask is provided, it is used to weight the loss and direct the network's focus towarddeformations in the tumor region. Consistent with the baseline, the first frame of each cine-MRI sequence is designated as the moving image, while all subsequent frames serve as fixed images. For each pair, the cumulative DVF warps the moving image to the fixed image and propagates the corresponding segmentation mask from the moving frame.

2.4 Training

In the unsupervised training phase, the objective was to learn inter-frame deformations between image pairs. To make training computationally feasible given the large volume of unlabeled data (2,863,827 frames), we sampled a reduced subset for unsupervised training, retaining sequences with clear anatomy, few artifacts, and regular organ-motion patterns. Regional annotations were omitted, and the model was trained for 200 epochs on an aggregated label-free dataset without distinction across anatomical regions. The total loss in the unsupervised training phase comprised two components: an image similarity loss, for MSE was used to ensure intensity consistency between the fixed image and the warped

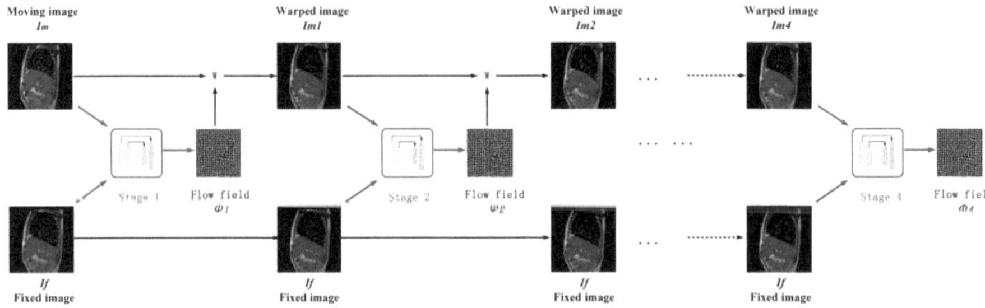

Fig. 1. Overview of the proposed C-VMorph network architecture.

moving image, and a deformation regularization loss, where the second derivative of the DVF was penalized as a bending energy term to encourage smooth deformations. The total loss can be expressed as a weighted sum of these terms:

$$\text{loss}_{\text{total}} = \gamma\, \text{loss}_{\text{img}} + \lambda\, \text{loss}_{\text{DVF}},$$

where γ was set to 1, and λ was set to 0.2. During the unsupervised phase, all available labeled data were reserved exclusively for validation. The Dice similarity coefficient was computed on this set after each epoch, and the model checkpoint with the highest Dice score was selected as the best unsupervised model.

The supervised training stage was initialized with the model weights obtained from the unsupervised training stage, and the labeled data were stratified by anatomies (pelvis, thorax, and abdomen). Because there are limited number of pelvic datasets, all available labeled data were used directly for training without a separate validation set. For the thoracic and abdominal sites, five labeled cases from each site were set aside for validation, and the remaining cases were used for training. Each site was trained for 200 epochs. In the supervised phase, the total loss function was extended to include Dice loss in addition to the image similarity and DVF regularization terms:

$$\text{loss}_{\text{total}} = \gamma\, \text{loss}_{\text{img}} + \lambda\, \text{loss}_{\text{DVF}} + \beta\, \text{loss}_{\text{Dice}},$$

where the weights for the image loss, DVF loss, and Dice loss were set to 1, 0.2, and 1, respectively.

We used the Adam optimizer with an initial learning rate of 1e-4. Additionally, the StepLR scheduler was employed, with a decay rate of 0.1 applied every 100 epochs. All training was conducted on a GeForce RTX 4090Ti 24GB GPU.

2.5 Post-Processing

In the post-processing step, morphological operations were applied to refine the output segmentation. Specifically, morphological opening followed by closing was performed using a 5×5 square structuring element, which effectively removed small noise, filled gaps, and smoothed the segmentation mask.

2.6 Evaluation

The model's segmentation performance was quantified against ground-truth labels using four geometric metrics and a radiotherapy-specific dosimetric index. Additionally, the inference time per cine-MRI frame was reported to demonstrate computational efficiency. A summary of the evaluation metrics is provided in Table 1.

3 Result

In the preliminary test phase, we evaluated our model on 8 cases, comprising 2 acquired with a 0.35 T MRI-linac and 6 with a 1.5 T MRI-linac. The mean results for the geometric, dosimetric, and runtime metrics are presented in Table 2.

Table 1. Evaluation metrics used for model performance assessment.

Evaluation type	Metrics	Description
Geometric metrics	Dice Similarity Coefficient (DSC)	Overlap between predicted and ground-truth segmentation
	Hausdorff Distance (HD95)	95th percentile of surface distances between predicted and ground-truth contours
	Mean Average Surface Distance (MASD)	Mean surface distance between predicted and ground-truth segmentations
	Center Distance (CD)	Euclidean distance between the centroids of the predicted and ground-truth segmentations
Dose metric	Dose accuracy	Accuracy of dose delivery with MLC tracking, evaluated by the relative D98% difference between ground-truth and shifted dose distributions
Runtime	Runtime per frame	Average inference time per cine-MRI frame

Table 2. Preliminary test results for geometric, dosimetric, and runtime metrics.

Model	Dice	CD (mm)	HD 95 (mm)	MASD (mm)	D98 dose
UTSRmorph	0.8786	2.2671	5.2806	1.8702	0.8724
cre C-VMorph	0.8990	2.0104	4.8004	1.6242	0.8715

As shown in Table 2, the four-iteration Cascade-VoxelMorph model (C-VMorph) consistently outperformed UTSRmorph in geometric accuracy, producing lower HD95 (4.8004 mm compared to 5.2806 mm) and MASD (1.6242 mm compared to 1.8702 mm), as well as a smaller center distance (2.0104 mm compared to 2.2671 mm). For the dosimetric evaluation, the two models achieved comparable results, with UTSRmorph showing a slightly higher D98 (0.8724 compared to 0.8715 for C-VMorph). Overall, these findings highlight the superior geometric alignment achieved by the cascaded CNN-based model, while maintaining comparable dose coverage relative to the transformer-based baseline.

In the final test phase, our four-iteration C-VMorph network was further evaluated on 50 cases (25 acquired at 0.35 T and 25 at 1.5 T), and the average results are reported in Table 3.

Table 3. Final test results of the four-iteration Cascade-VoxelMorph network.

Model	Dice	CD (mm)	HD 95 (mm)	MASD (mm)	D98 dose	Runtime (ms/frame)
C-VMorph	0.8510	2.3009	5.3346	2.2996	0.9078	55.3

4 Discussion

The results demonstrate that the C-VMorph network provided superior geometric accuracy compared with UTSRmorph, while achieving comparable dose coverage and per-frame runtime. This performance difference may be attributed to the larger parameterization of UTSRmorph's hybrid Transformer-CNN architecture, which increases susceptibility to overfitting under limited training data and can restrict generalization to unseen cine-MRI sequences. In contrast, the cascaded CNN design of the C-VMorph, with iterative refinement across four stages, leading to more stable deformation fields for tumor tracking.

Building on these findings, several promising directions remain for future research. First, while Transformer-based models such as UTSRmorph effectively capture long-range dependencies, their large parameter counts increase the risk of overfitting and impose substantial computational demands. Future work could integrate selected Transformer modules into cascaded CNN frameworks to balance global context modeling with computational efficiency. Second, although this study employed a four-iteration cascade to trade off accuracy and runtime, techniques such as model distillation or adaptive iteration scheduling may further reduce inference cost without compromising accuracy, making the approach more practical for real-time deployment. Finally, instead of training on the full dataset, we adopted a sampling strategy to manage efficiency. Future efforts could explore more systematic data selection methods to ensure that sampled cases remain maximally representative, thereby allowing the model to capture a broader range of anatomical and motion variability without substantially increasing training cost.

5 Conclusion

In this study, we compared a C-VMorph network with a Transformer-CNN baseline (UTSRmorph) for real-time 2D tumor tracking in cine-MRI. Despite having fewer parameters and lower complexity, the C-VMorph achieved performance comparable to the baseline. These findings suggest that lightweight CNN-based architectures offer a practical and efficient alternative for MRI-guided radiotherapy under real-time constraints. Future work will focus on further improving tracking accuracy and efficiency through architectural refinements.

References

1. Hall, W.A., Paulson, E.S., van der Heide, U.A., et al.: The transformation of radiation oncology using real-time magnetic resonance guidance: a review. Eur. J. Cancer **122**, 42–52 (2019)
2. Kurz, C., Buizza, G., Landry, G., et al.: Medical physics challenges in clinical MR-guided radiotherapy. Radiat. Oncol. **15**(1), 93 (2020)
3. Keall, P.J., Glide-Hurst, C.K., Cao, M., et al.: ICRU REPORT 97: MRI-guided radiation therapy using MRI-linear accelerators. J. ICRU **22**(1), 1–100 (2022)
4. Grimbergen, G., Hackett, S. L., van Ommen, F., et al.: Gating and intrafraction drift correction on a 1.5 T MR-Linac: clinical dosimetric benefits for upper abdominal tumors. Radiother. Oncol. **189**, 109932 (2023)
5. Liu, P.Z.Y., Dong, B., Nguyen, D.T., et al.: First experimental investigation of simultaneously tracking two independently moving targets on an MRI-linac using real-time MRI and MLC tracking. Med. Phys. **47**(12), 6440–6449 (2020)
6. Lombardo, E., Liu, P.Z.Y., Waddington, D.E.J., et al.: Experimental comparison of linear regression and LSTM motion prediction models for MLC-tracking on an MRI-linac. Med. Phys. **50**(11), 7083–7092 (2023)
7. Shi, X., Diwanji, T., Mooney, K.E., et al.: Evaluation of template matching for tumor motion management with cine-MR images in lung cancer patients. Med. Phys. **41**(5), 052304 (2014)
8. Keiper, T.D., Tai, A., Chen, X., et al.: Feasibility of real-time motion tracking using cine MRI during MR-guided radiation therapy for abdominal targets. Med. Phys. **47**(8), 3554–3566 (2020)
9. Jassar, H., Tai, A., Chen, X.: Real-time motion monitoring using orthogonal cine MRI during MR-guided adaptive radiation therapy for abdominal tumors on 1.5 T MR-Linac. Med. Phys. **50**(5), 3103–3116 (2023)
10. Fast, M.F., Eiben, B., Menten, M.J., et al.: Tumour auto-contouring on 2D cine MRI for locally advanced lung cancer: a comparative study. Radiother. Oncol. **125**(3), 485–491 (2017)
11. Palacios, M.A., Gerganov, G., Cobussen, P., et al.: Accuracy of deformable image registration-based intra-fraction motion management in Magnetic Resonance-guided radiotherapy. Phys. Imaging Radiat. Oncol. **26**, 100437 (2023)
12. Feng, Y., Kawrakow, I., Olsen, J., et al.: A comparative study of automatic image segmentation algorithms for target tracking in MR-IGRT. J. Appl. Clin. Med. Phys. **17**(2), 441–460 (2016)
13. Blöcker, T., Lombardo, E., Marschner, S.N., et al.: MRgRT real-time target localization using foundation models for contour point tracking and promptable mask refinement. Phys. Med. Biol. **70**(1), 015004 (2024)

14. Lombardo, E., Velezmoro, L., Marschner, S.N., et al.: Patient-specific deep learning tracking framework for real-time 2D target localization in magnetic resonance imaging-guided radiation therapy. Int. J. Radiat. Oncol. Biol. Phys. **122**(4), 827–837 (2025)
15. Zhang, R., Mo, H., Wang, J.: UTSRMorph: a unified transformer and superresolution network for unsupervised medical image registration. IEEE Trans. Med. Imaging (2024)
16. Balakrishnan, G., Zhao, A., Sabuncu, M.R., et al.: VoxelMorph: a learning framework for deformable medical image registration. IEEE Trans. Med. Imaging **38**(8), 1788–1800 (2019)
17. Wang, Y., Lombardo, E., Thummerer, A., et al.: TrackRAD2025 challenge dataset: real-time tumor tracking for MRI-guided radiotherapy. Med. Phys. **52**(7), e17964 (2025)

Boundary-Aware Deformable Registration for MRI-Guided Radiotherapy

Konstantinos Georgas(✉), Theodoros P. Vagenas, and George K. Matsopoulos

Biomedical Engineering Lab (BEL), School of Electrical and Computer Engineering, National Technical University of Athens, 15780 Athens, Greece
{kostasgeo,tpvagenas,gmatsopoulos}@biomed.ntua.gr
https://www.biomed.ntua.gr/

Abstract. Magnetic Resonance Imaging (MRI) is an essential component of current cancer treatment systems for imaging interior anatomical structures. However, accurate real-time tumour segmentation for adaptive radiation therapy is complicated by tissue motion and deformation. Precise registration is often challenging for standard imaging registration algorithms due to large displacement errors and the need for real-time application in clinical settings. This challenge is further intensified for accurate real-time tracking algorithms used in cancer therapy. For the proposed application involving real-time tumor tracking using the 2D cine-MRI technique and a deep learning approach for deformable image registration tasks with the enhanced TransMorph model, the model has been designed to include attention gates in the skip connections of the decoder. Additionally, the approach employs a two-step robust learning process: the first step involves unsupervised learning from patient image data to capture generic deformation information. To ensure boundary accuracy, a combined loss function method has been adopted, comprising boundary-weighted Dice loss, Adaptive Mean-Squared Error (MSE) loss with L1 regularizer, Smooth-Diffusion loss, and Edge loss. Validated on the multi-institutional TrackRAD2025 dataset, the proposed framework consistently outperformed baseline transformer-based models in both overlap metrics and boundary error reduction. These results highlight the potential of the attention-guided framework to enable accurate, real-time tumor tracking in MRI-guided radiotherapy.

Keywords: Real-Time MRI · Adaptive Radiotherapy · Non-rigid Registration · Hierarchical Vision Transformer · Spatial Attention · Tumor Tracking

1 Introduction

The advent of Magnetic Resonance-guided Radiotherapy (MRgRT) systems represents a paradigm shift in the delivery of oncological therapies, as they provide

J. P. Wachs et al. (Eds.): TrackRAD/TTC 2025, LNCS 16474, pp. 61–69, 2027.
https://doi.org/10.1007/978-3-032-35046-6_7

non-invasive and high-contrast visualization of soft tissue targets during irradiation [7]. Unlike Cone Beam CT scanners, the potential of MR linacs lies in their ability to monitor anatomical changes in real time, offering a possible solution to the longstanding problem of managing intrafraction motion uncertainties [12]. However, the real-time functionality of these machines creates a significant computational challenge: the need to achieve subcycle resolution tumor tracking to enable breathing or MLC tracking [4].

Currently, this process relies on optimization-driven Deformable Image Registration (DIR) or template matching. Although highly accurate, these iterative approaches often exhibited high latency, making them unsuitable for the millisecond response times required in clinical applications. Consequently, there has been a paradigm shift towards Deep Learning (DL)-based methods, which transfer most computation to an offline training environment, enabling nearly instantaneous processing. Although early Convolutional Neural Networks (CNNs), such as VoxelMorph, demonstrated the conceptual feasibility of unsupervised approaches [1], they have been shown to possess short receptive fields, making this strategy suboptimal for managing long-range deformations, as seen in organ motion in the abdominal or chest regions [13].

To address these limitations, the field of medical imaging has recently seen the application of Vision Transformers (ViTs), which incorporate self-attention mechanisms to handle global relations learned from the entire image volume [6]. Hierarchical approaches, including Swin Transformers and, more recently, H-ViT, have achieved outstanding results by efficiently combining features at various scales [5]. Nevertheless, local feature representation may still be problematic in exclusively Transformer-based approaches for image registration. This is because, during patch-merging operations required to increase the size of the receptive field, high-frequency spatial information, especially that involving tumor borders, is likely to be lost in the process [6,15]. In the proposed study, a TransMorph framework [2] with integrated attention mechanisms is presented to bridge the gap between global motion modeling and the fulfillment of boundary requirements. It is assumed that despite the fact that the Swin Transformer architecture successfully addresses global motion modeling and achieves efficient anatomical transformation modeling, the decoding component requires additional spatial attention gates to accurately capture tumor boundary information. By strategically integrating attention gates into the skip connections of a suitably modified TransMorph architecture, the proposed framework enables the network to filter out background noise and highlight highly relevant information. This approach was evaluated using the TrackRAD2025 benchmark dataset [17], which demonstrates the efficacy of the attention mechanism in achieving enhanced tracking and boundary performance while preserving the necessary real-time processing speed.

2 Methods

2.1 Data Cohort and Acquisition Protocols

The TrackRAD2025 dataset [17], containing 108 labeled and 477 unlabeled sagittal cine-MRI sequences from six global centers, was employed. Tumors from thoracic, abdominal, and pelvic regions were included, imaged at 0.35 T or 1.5 T, each with a tumor mask on the first frame. Training utilized the full public cohort (477 unlabeled, 50 labeled cases). Hyperparameters were tuned on 10 labeled cases, with the remaining 40 used for supervised training. Unlabeled cases were used solely for pretraining.

2.2 Data Harmonization and Augmentation Strategy

Given the differences in acquisition parameters (e.g., gain, resolution, and field of view), a robust method for data harmonization was implemented to reduce domain shifts. Inspired by the self-configuring paradigm proposed in the nnU-Net architecture [8], the z-scoring on a per-patient basis was adopted to normalize the intensity values for each frame. To account for scanner-dependent contrast differences, histogram matching was performed between the reference frame and the dynamic frames to equalize the intensity values. To promote invariance to anatomical variations and imaging artifacts, a comprehensive online augmentation strategy was implemented [3]. Spatial invariance was encouraged through random affine perturbations, specifically rotation ($\pm 15°$), translation (± 10 px), and shear (± 0.05). Additionally, robustness to image quality degradation was addressed by simulating bias field inhomogeneities, Gibbs ringing artifacts, and Gaussian blurring. The dataset was subsequently divided into an 80/20 split for training and evaluation.

2.3 Model Architecture

Spatially-Gated TransMorph framework is presented, a hierarchical architecture that combines the long-range dependency learning capability of the Transformer architecture with the localization required for cancer tracking tasks. A high-level overview of this system is shown in Fig. 1.

The backbone is based on Swin Transformer modules [11], which use shifted window self-attention to generate multi-scale features $\{f_1, f_2, f_3, f_4\}$. Although these modules are highly effective at capturing global deformation patterns, downsampling is required to increase the receptive field size, which can reduce local, detailed, high-frequency patterns. Spatial Gating Units are used as bridges between encoders and decoders to compensate for potential losses due to downsampling. A learned saliency for gating irrelevant background patterns may improve attributes related to peripheral areas around tumors [14].

The formal expression for the gating function is:

$$\alpha = \sigma\big(W^{\top} \operatorname{ReLU}(W_g g + W_x x + b)\big) \tag{1}$$

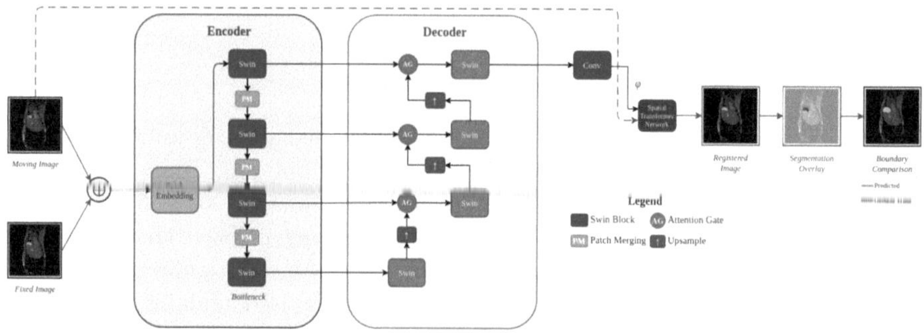

Fig. 1. Overview of the proposed registration network architecture. The model extends TransMorph standard architecture [2] by incorporating attention-gated skip connections to selectively propagate spatially relevant features during decoding. The encoder uses a hierarchical Swin-Transformer backbone with patch merging operations to extract multi-scale feature representations. These features are passed to the decoder through attention gates (AG), which learn to emphasize salient spatial regions while suppressing irrelevant background information. The decoder progressively upsamples the feature maps and fuses them with attention-weighted encoder features at corresponding resolution levels. A convolutional layer generates the dense deformation field ϕ, which is then applied to the moving image via a spatial transformer network to produce the registered output. The architecture supports both supervised training with segmentation guidance (3-channel input) and unsupervised training (2-channel input).

where g is the gating signal from the coarse-scale decoder, x represents the features from the skip connections, and σ denotes the sigmoid activation function. These gated features, $\hat{x}$, are then integrated into the decoder path. Ultimately, a deformation field ϕ is produced using a convolutional head with a spatial transformer module [9]. The network contains approximately 31 million parameters, with Xavier uniform initialization.

2.4 Optimization Framework and Loss Functions

A dual-stage curriculum learning framework was adopted to optimize network parameters θ to ensure topological regularity and accurate segmentation.

Phase I: Unsupervised Regularization. The model was pre-trained on the unlabeled set (477 sequences) to learn an initial representation of general anatomical motion. This step aimed to jointly minimize an objective combining image similarity and smoothness: $L_{unsup} = \lambda_{MSE}||T(I_m, \phi) - I_{target}||_2^2 + \lambda_{smooth}L_{smooth}$ where L_{smooth} regularizes the spatial gradients of the displacement field towards diffeomorphism-like mappings and I_m denotes the moving image.

Phase II: Boundary-Aware Fine-Tuning. In the supervised learning phase, the model was fine-tuned on the labeled subset using a loss function designed to penalize misalignments in the boundary region. The total loss function was defined as: $L_{sup} = \lambda_{im} L_1 + \lambda_{edge} ||E(I_{target}) - E(T(I_m, \phi))||_1 + \lambda_{Dice} L_{DSC}$ where $E(\cdot)$ is a Sobel-based edge extraction operator. This specific edge alignment term encourages the network to align structural boundaries, which often have low contrast in cine-MRI images. In addition, a Dice loss function with a weighted boundary was used to promote precise overlap of the tumor area with the background.

2.5 Performance Evaluation Metrics

For quantitative analysis, metrics assessing both volume overlap and geometric accuracy were used. The Dice Similarity Coefficient (DSC) was selected as the primary metric for overlap calculation. To address the need for boundary accuracy, particularly in radiotherapy margin definition, the 95th percentile Hausdorff Distance (HD95) and the Median Hausdorff Distance (HD50) were calculated. Inference time was also measured to evaluate potential use in real-time applications. Significance testing was performed using the Wilcoxon signed-rank test with alpha < 0.05 [18].

3 Results

3.1 Model Performance

Table 1 provides a comparative analysis of the proposed framework against the baseline TransMorph model and its ablative variants. Performance in the validation cohort is reported on five metrics to offer a comprehensive assessment of both volumetric overlap and geometric boundary fidelity. The introduction of the hybrid loss function alone yielded a marginal increase in the Dice Similarity Coefficient (DSC); however, it significantly improved boundary precision, reducing the 95% Hausdorff Distance (95HD) from 4.24 mm to 3.87 mm. This suggests that the explicit edge-alignment terms in the loss function effectively enhance the model's sensitivity to structural interfaces.

The incorporation of attention gates into skip connections further refined the accuracy of the registration. The complete proposed framework, integrating both the spatial gating mechanism and the hybrid loss, outperformed all baseline configurations. In particular, it achieved a state-of-the-art DSC of **0.9342**, while substantially minimizing the 95HD to **2.75 mm** and the Median Hausdorff Distance (50HD) to **0.88 mm**. An increase in the negative Jacobian determinant ($J\phi < 0$) was observed, likely indicating that the model permits more complex, non-linear local deformations to maximize alignment accuracy. Crucially, this performance gain was achieved without compromising computational efficiency; the mean inference time remained approximately **24.70 ms**, validating the model's suitability for real-time tracking applications. Statistical significance

Table 1. Validation performance on the TrackRAD2025 validation set. All values are reported as mean ± standard deviation.

Method	DSC↑	95HD↓	50HD↓	NEGJ↓	Time (ms)↓
Base (Transmorph)	0.9151±0.06	4.24±6.19	1.51±2.48	**1.95±0.98**	23.70±8.90
Base + Hybrid loss	0.9167±0.06	3.87±4.80	1.25±1.73	4.79±3.15	**23.30±8.20**
Base + Attention	0.9203±0.06	3.90±5.92	1.34±2.13	4.62±1.80	25.20±8.30
Proposed	**0.9342±0.05**	**2.75±3.24**	**0.88±0.40**	5.36±3.69	24.70±8.00

in improving DSC was confirmed for the proposed method compared to baseline variants ($p < 0.05$).

Figure 2 depicts a baseline segmentation outcome on cine-MRI frames. The warped image is the result of the suggested model, demonstrating that the moving image was precisely aligned with the fixed image. The model indicates remarkable alignment, with a significant overlap between the predicted and actual tumor masks. The matching flow image further shows that the model emphasizes on the tumor location throughout the alignment procedure.

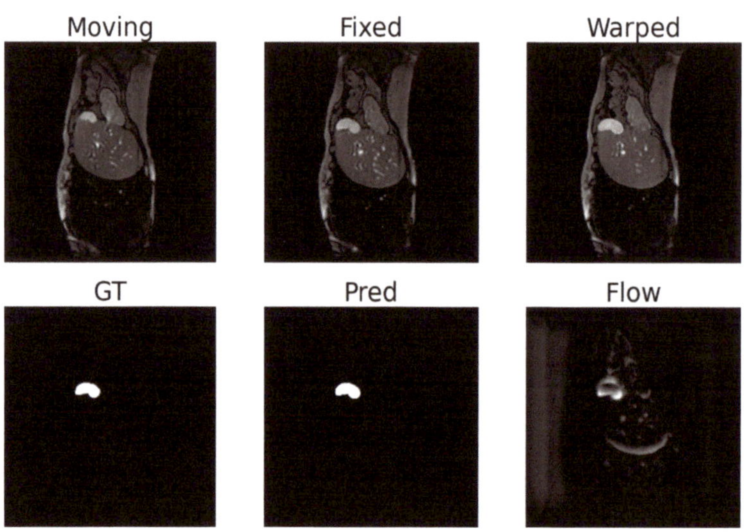

Fig. 2. Qualitative example showing successful tumor tracking. **Top row:** Moving image, Fixed image, and Warped (registered) image. **Bottom row:** Ground truth segmentation (GT), Predicted segmentation (Pred), and corresponding deformation flow field (Flow).

4 Discussion

The empirical findings in this study support the potential of Transformer-based architectures to overcome the latency-accuracy trade-off inherent in real-time image guidance. By expanding the global receptive field of the Swin Transformer with spatially gated attention mechanisms, the proposed framework effectively filters background noise and prioritizes salient tumor features during inference. Additionally, the integration of hybrid supervision – specifically, the combination of boundary-aware loss functions and motion-oriented augmentations – significantly contributes to maintaining segmentation fidelity. This synergy is especially effective in addressing the low-contrast soft-tissue interfaces and dynamic anatomical shifts that characterize cine-MRI acquisitions.

Despite these promising outcomes, several methodological constraints require critical consideration. A primary limitation of the current framework is its reliance on independent 2D frame processing. By treating the cine-MRI sequence as a collection of disjoint snapshots, the model overlooks the inherent temporal coherence and physiological continuity of the respiratory cycle. This lack of temporal context may compromise tracking stability during phases of rapid anatomical displacement or irregular breathing patterns, potentially introducing high-frequency jitter in the estimated trajectory. Future investigations could address this by incorporating recurrent neural networks (RNNs) or sequence-aware spatiotemporal modules [10] to explicitly model the temporal dependencies of organ motion.

Additionally, the network's generalization capabilities may be limited by the distributional characteristics of the training cohort. The dataset used in this study is heavily skewed toward specific anatomical regions (predominantly thoracic) and magnetic field strengths (0.35 and 1.5 T). Such imbalances can cause domain overfitting, making it difficult for the model to adapt to the signal-to-noise ratios or contrast profiles of underrepresented acquisition protocols. To improve clinical robustness, future work could explore unsupervised domain adaptation techniques or multi-source feature alignment strategies [16] to reduce the impact of inter-institutional variability.

Finally, regarding the statistical rigor of the validation, the relatively limited size of the labeled validation set constrained the power of formal hypothesis testing in this analysis. While reporting uncertainty estimates across validation folds indicates model stability, the current assessment relies primarily on descriptive performance metrics. Subsequent benchmarking with larger, statistically independent test cohorts will be necessary to rigorously quantify the significance of the observed performance gains relative to competing state-of-the-art methods.

Author contributions. The authors declare contributions in accordance with the CRediT (Contributor Roles Taxonomy):

- **Konstantinos Georgas (PhD Candidate)**: Conceptualization; Methodology; Software; Validation; Formal Analysis; Investigation; Resources; Data Curation; Writing – Original Draft; Writing – Review & Editing; Visualization; Writing – Review & Editing.

– **Theodoros P. Vagenas (PhD Candidate)**: Conceptualization; Methodology; Software; Validation; Formal Analysis; Investigation; Resources; Data Curation; Writing – Original Draft; Writing – Review & Editing; Visualization; Writing – Review & Editing.
– **Prof. George K. Matsopoulos**: Supervision; Project Administration.

Other Information. The authors state that there was no external funding or institutional collaboration that contributed to this work. There are no competing interests.

References

1. Balakrishnan, G., Zhao, A., Sabuncu, M.R., Guttag, J., Dalca, A.V.: VoxelMorph: a learning framework for deformable medical image registration. IEEE Trans. Med. Imaging **38**(8), 1788–1800 (2019). https://doi.org/10.1109/TMI.2019.2897538
2. Chen, J., et al.: TransMorph: transformer for unsupervised medical image registration. Med. Image Anal. **82**, 102615 (2022). https://doi.org/10.1016/j.media.2022.102615
3. Chlap, P., et al.: A review of medical image data augmentation techniques for deep learning applications. J. Med. Imaging Radiat. Oncol. **65**(5), 545–563 (2021). https://doi.org/10.1111/1754-9485.13261
4. Eiben, B., et al.: Respiratory motion modelling for MR-guided lung cancer radiotherapy: model development and geometric accuracy evaluation. Phys. Med. Biol. **69**(6), 065009 (2024). https://doi.org/10.1088/1361-6560/ad222f
5. Ghahremani, M.: H-ViT: a hierarchical vision transformer for deformable image registration. In: Proceedings of the IEEE/CVF Conference on Computer Vision and Pattern Recognition (CVPR), pp. 11513–11523 (2024)
6. Henry, E.U., et al.: Vision transformers in medical imaging: a review. Med. Image Anal. **91**, 103000 (2024). https://doi.org/10.1016/j.media.2023.103000
7. Herrera, R.A., et al.: Evolving trends and patterns of utilization of magnetic resonance-guided radiotherapy at a single institution, 2018–2024. Cancers **17**(2), 208 (2025). https://doi.org/10.3390/cancers17020208
8. Isensee, F., et al.: nnU-Net: a self-configuring method for deep learning-based biomedical image segmentation. Nat. Methods **18**(2), 203–211 (2021). https://doi.org/10.1038/s41592-020-01008-z
9. Jaderberg, M., Simonyan, K., Zisserman, A., Kavukcuoglu, K.: Spatial transformer networks. In: Cortes, C., Lawrence, N.D., Lee, D.D., Sugiyama, M., Garnett, R. (eds.) Advances in Neural Information Processing Systems, vol. 28, pp. 2017–2025. Curran Associates, Inc., Red Hook (2015). https://doi.org/10.48550/arXiv.1506.02025
10. Li, Z., et al.: Temporally consistent motion estimation for cine MRI using temporal regularization and transformer networks. In: Wang, L., et al. (eds.) Medical Image Computing and Computer Assisted Intervention – MICCAI 2022, pp. 294–304. Springer, Cham (2022). https://doi.org/10.1007/978-3-031-16443-9_29
11. Liu, Z., et al.: Swin transformer: hierarchical vision transformer using shifted windows. In: Proceedings of the IEEE/CVF International Conference on Computer Vision (ICCV), pp. 10012–10022 (2021). https://doi.org/10.1109/ICCV48922.2021.00986
12. Lombardo, E.: Deep learning for real-time motion management during MRI-guided radiotherapy. Dissertation, LMU Munich (2025). https://doi.org/10.5282/edoc.35836

13. Ma, J., et al.: Rethinking the effective receptive field in deep learning for medical image segmentation. IEEE Trans. Med. Imaging (2024). https://doi.org/10.1109/TMI.2024.3366776
14. Oktay, O., et al.: Attention U-net: learning where to look for the pancreas. arXiv preprint arXiv:1804.03999 (2018). https://doi.org/10.48550/arXiv.1804.03999
15. Shamshad, F., et al.: Transformers in medical imaging: a survey. Med. Image Anal. **88**, 102802 (2023). https://doi.org/10.1016/j.media.2023.102802
16. Valindria, V.V., et al.: Multi-modal learning from unpaired images: application to multi-organ segmentation in CT and MRI. In: Proceedings of the IEEE Conference on Computer Vision and Pattern Recognition (CVPR) Workshops, pp. 2485–2494 (2018). https://doi.org/10.1109/CVPRW.2018.00318
17. Wang, Y.: TrackRAD2025 challenge dataset: real-time tumor tracking for MRI-guided radiotherapy. arXiv preprint arXiv:2503.19119 (2025)
18. Wilcoxon, F.: Individual comparisons by ranking methods. Biomet. Bull. **1**(6), 80–83 (1945). https://doi.org/10.2307/3001968

The Trauma THOMPSON Challenge 2025

Overview of the Trauma THOMPSON Challenge at MICCAI 2025

Yupeng Zhuo[1], Eddie Zhang[1], Xiangchen Yu[1], Aditya Pachpande[1], Andrew W. Kirkpatrick[2], Jessica McKee[2], Edgar Rojas-Muñoz[3], Brian VanVoorst[4], Jin Tae Kwak[5], Stas Tiomkin[6], Yanjun Gao[7], and Juan P. Wachs[1(✉)]

[1] Purdue University, West Lafayette, IN, USA
jpwachs@purdue.edu
[2] University of Calgary, Calgary, AB, Canada
[3] Texas A&M University, College Station, TX, USA
[4] RTX BBN Technologies, Cambridge, MA, USA
[5] Korea University, Seoul, South Korea
[6] Texas Tech University, Lubbock, TX, USA
[7] University of Colorado Anschutz Medical Campus, Aurora, CO, USA

Abstract. The Trauma THOMPSON Challenge 2025 aims to advance autonomous systems capable of providing real-time procedural guidance in resource-constrained and austere environments. Utilizing a comprehensive egocentric dataset of 3,717 unscripted medical sequences captured by head-mounted cameras, the challenge encompasses five clinically relevant tasks: action recognition and anticipation, hand tracking, tool detection, realism assessment, and visual question answering. A key innovation in this iteration is the inclusion of "just-in-time" (JIT) procedures that utilize improvised daily objects, such as belts and screwdrivers, to evaluate model generalizability under unpredictable field conditions. Active participation was observed in three tasks, with performance in action recognition showing a significant leap from the 35.27% top-1 accuracy recorded in the 2023 challenge to a new benchmark of 61.48%. Top-performing methodologies integrated spatiotemporal 3D convolutional neural networks with temporal modeling and data-centric object detection frameworks. Despite these advancements, the JIT procedures and complex surgical backgrounds remain substantial hurdles, with tasks such as tool detection and VQA receiving no submissions due to specialized infrastructure requirements. These findings underscore the potential of medical foundation models and temporal modeling while highlighting the ongoing need for domain-independent learning to ensure operational reliability in humanitarian and battlefield medicine.

Keywords: Deep learning · Action recognition · Action anticipation · Just-in-time procedures · Hand tracking · Object detection · Realism assessment · Visual question answering

---

Disclaimers: The views, opinions, and/or findings contained in this report are those of the author(s) and should not be construed as an official Department of the Army position, policy, or decision unless so designated by other documentation.

J. P. Wachs et al. (Eds.): TrackRAD/TTC 2025, LNCS 16474, pp. 73–91, 2027.
https://doi.org/10.1007/978-3-032-35046-6_8

1 Introduction

The increasing frequency of global pandemics and regional conflicts has amplified the demand for autonomous systems capable of delivering real time medical guidance in resource constrained environments. Such systems are especially critical in austere or uncontrolled settings where conventional medical infrastructure is either severely compromised or entirely absent [1]. In these contexts, medical personnel often face the dual challenge of navigating difficult terrain while managing complex trauma cases over extended periods with limited support [2,3]. Given that a large proportion of trauma related deaths occur within the so called golden hour before patients reach advanced care facilities, the ability to provide timely and accurate intervention at the point of injury is a decisive factor in patient survival [4].

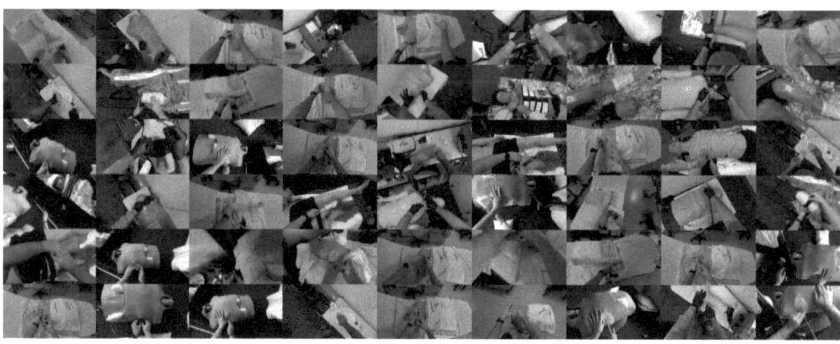

Fig. 1. Examples of Trauma THOMPSON procedures.

The Trauma TeleHelper for Operational Medical Procedure Support and Offline Network (Trauma THOMPSON) Challenge introduces a comprehensive dataset designed to advance the development of autonomous medical instruction systems for emergency care in low resource settings [5,6], as shown in Fig. 1. The envisioned system is capable of recognizing ongoing actions, predicting subsequent steps, tracking hand movements, detecting and highlighting medical tools, and answering medically relevant queries. Such functionality enables the system to assist inexperienced providers by offering critical procedural guidance and contextual information. The dataset includes professionally annotated video sequences with high quality bounding boxes for hands and tools, realism scores, and frame level visual question answering (VQA) annotations. Notably, it represents one of the first large scale egocentric datasets capturing unscripted medical procedures across diverse and realistic environments. The data are collected from medical experts performing emergency interventions on highly realistic simulators, as well as just in time procedures that utilize tools of daily life. These scenarios reflect real world conditions where standard equipment may not be available but immediate intervention remains essential.

Each video is annotated with ground truth actions represented as verb noun pairs, along with temporal boundaries that define the duration of each action. This representation improves interpretability by explicitly linking actions to their targets [7]. Additional annotations include hand trajectories, object detections, and realism scores, all of which provide valuable context for understanding procedural dynamics. The unscripted nature of the recorded procedures ensures that the dataset closely reflects the variability and unpredictability encountered in real humanitarian settings. Furthermore, each clip is associated with a specific life saving skill, reinforcing the dataset's relevance to critical care scenarios. Collectively, these characteristics establish the dataset as a significant resource for advancing research in autonomous medical assistance and improving procedural outcomes in challenging environments [6].

The first Trauma THOMPSON Challenge was organized as a satellite event at Medical Image Computing and Computer Assisted Intervention (MICCAI) 2023 and featured two tracks comprising four tasks [5]. These included action recognition, action anticipation, procedure classification, and VQA. The action recognition task focused on identifying actions within egocentric video sequences using temporal annotations, while action anticipation required predicting future steps in a procedure. Procedure recognition aimed to classify the overall type of intervention, and the VQA task evaluated the ability of models to interpret both visual and textual inputs to answer clinically relevant questions. The dataset for this initial challenge consisted of several hundred annotated videos covering five essential life saving procedures, including cricothyroidotomy, intraosseous infusion, needle thoracostomy, tourniquet application, and tube thoracostomy.

The second iteration of the Trauma THOMPSON Challenge expands both the dataset and the scope of tasks, introducing five distinct challenges that reflect more complex and realistic scenarios. The first task combines action recognition and anticipation within a unified framework, requiring models to simultaneously interpret current actions and predict future steps. The second and third tasks focus on hand tracking and tool detection, respectively, both of which are essential for monitoring procedural execution and ensuring correct instrument usage. The fourth task introduces realism assessment, which evaluates the fidelity of simulated procedures and can inform training strategies for improving model generalization. The fifth task extends VQA by incorporating more complex queries that require deeper contextual reasoning beyond direct visual cues.

These tasks are carefully designed to align with the requirements of real time telementoring systems, where accurate perception, prediction, and interaction are essential. Action recognition and anticipation enable timely guidance, particularly in high pressure environments where rapid decision making is critical. The inclusion of just in time procedures introduces additional complexity due to the use of improvised tools and the absence of standardized workflows, thereby increasing the variability that models must handle. Realism assessment contributes to improving the training process by prioritizing data that better reflects real world conditions. Hand tracking supports skill evaluation by analyzing motion patterns, while tool detection ensures that appropriate instruments are identified and utilized. Overall, the second challenge presents a more demanding and practically relevant benchmark, emphasizing the development of robust systems capable of operating effectively in real world emergency scenarios.

2 Task 1: Action Recognition and Anticipation of Regular and Just in-Time Procedures

2.1 Datasets

Data Sources. The procedure videos were captured from an egocentric perspective using head-mounted cameras, specifically a GoPro Hero 7 or higher. This device supports high-resolution video recording in MP4 format with elevated frame rates, enabling precise visual representation of medical procedures. To enhance dataset diversity, recordings were conducted across a range of environments.

Data collection protocols were adapted from the EPIC-KITCHENS benchmark [7]. Cameras were mounted on the heads of participants to ensure a first-person viewpoint during procedural execution. The recordings were performed in controlled settings designed to simulate field conditions, with an emphasis on procedures carried out by military medics and experienced medical professionals. Each video documents the real-time use of medical instruments.

Standardized imaging protocols were implemented to maintain data quality, including controlled lighting conditions to minimize shadows, ensure clear visibility of tools, and preserve consistent camera orientation across recordings. All videos were stored in MP4 format and subsequently annotated with temporal timestamps. In addition, frame-level data were extracted from the videos. Both annotated video sequences and corresponding frame data are provided as part of the dataset.

The data collection process involved trained military medics and medical professionals with substantial expertise in the documented procedures. Contributors included personnel affiliated with Purdue University, The Geneva Foundation, Madigan Army Medical Center, the Ready Medic One Research Team, and the University of Calgary. All participating physicians possessed over ten years of clinical experience. During recording, participants adjusted the head-mounted cameras to optimize viewpoint alignment, ensuring that hand movements remained centered within the frame throughout the procedures.

Training and Test Case Characteristics. The training and testing sets comprise video clips depicting procedures performed by military medics and experienced medical professionals. Each training instance includes a video clip accompanied by comprehensive annotations, including the current action, the subsequent action, and the corresponding start and end timestamps. Actions are represented as verbnoun pairs, consistent with standard formulations in egocentric action recognition. In contrast, each testing instance consists solely of a video clip without accompanying annotations.

The dataset contains a total of 3,717 instances, of which 2,930 samples (80%) are allocated for training and 787 samples (20%) for testing. This partitioning follows conventional practices in machine learning to ensure a balanced evaluation protocol. Participants may further subdivide the training set into training and validation subsets as required.

Although the dataset exhibits class imbalance, the distribution reflects real-world procedural frequencies. For regular procedures, the dataset includes 42 verb classes, 42 noun classes, and 124 distinct action classes, as illustrated in Fig. 2. For just-in-time (JIT) procedures, it comprises 28 verb classes, 32 noun classes, and 89 action classes, as illustrated in Fig. 3. These scenarios involved improvised medical tools, which contributed to a pronounced performance gap as models struggled to generalize beyond the regular procedures provided in the training data, as shown in Fig. 4.

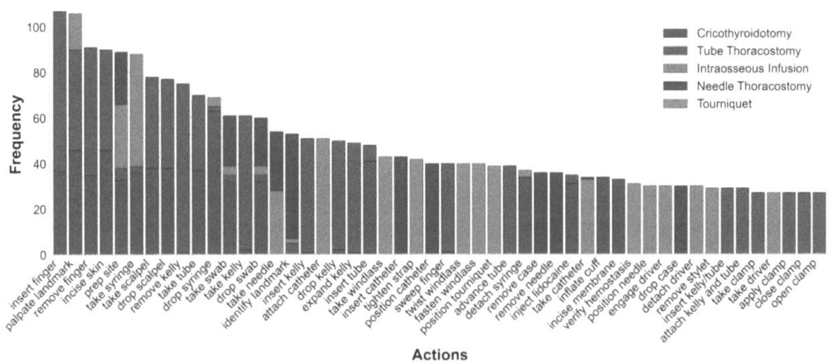

Fig. 2. Top 50 most frequent actions of regular procedures.

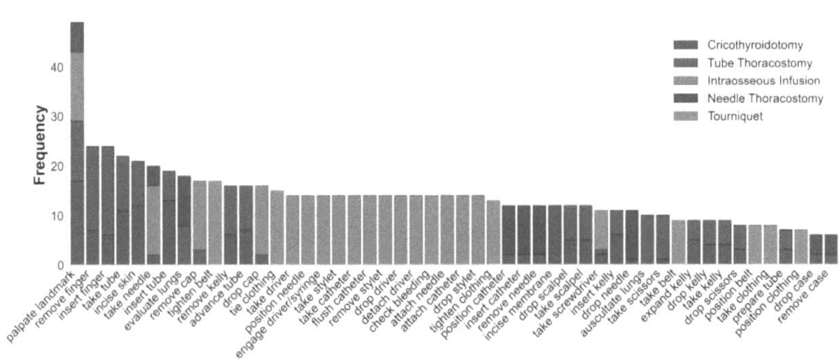

Fig. 3. Top 50 most frequent actions JIT procedures.

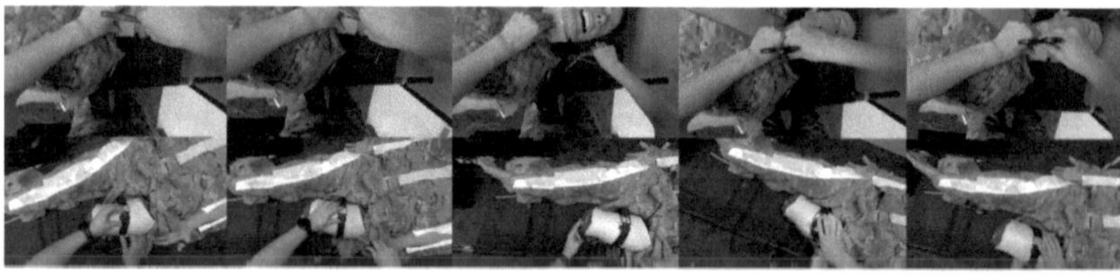

Fig. 4. Examples of JIT procedures.

Annotation Characteristics. Annotations include start and end timestamps, as well as labels for both current and subsequent actions within each video clip. The expected output for the test set consists of action, verb, and noun predictions. Following data collection, physicians annotated their own recordings by providing timestamps, action labels, and questionanswer pairs describing procedural steps. A total of five human annotators participated in the annotation and review process.

Annotation guidelines were established to ensure consistency. All annotations were required to be in present tense and formatted as verbnoun pairs (e.g., "incise skin", "take needle"), without the use of pronouns. Annotators were instructed to avoid including any identifying information to preserve privacy. For actions with extended duration, multiple annotations with identical labels but different timestamps were permitted. For example, a prolonged action such as "palpate landmark" could be segmented into multiple annotated intervals.

All annotators had over five years of medical experience. Each video clip is associated with a single, definitive annotation, eliminating ambiguity from multiple label sources. Following annotation, preprocessing was performed to standardize labels. Action descriptions were decomposed into verb and noun components, and semantically similar terms were grouped into unified classes (e.g., "pick" and "take" were consolidated into a single verb category).

2.2 Assessment Aim

The task of action recognition and anticipation in medical procedures challenges participants to simultaneously recognize current actions and predict next actions on egocentric medical procedure videos. This dual-task formulation closely mirrors real-world scenarios and needs in emergency medicine, battlefield medicine, and disaster response, where accurate and timely interpretation of medical actions is crucial for effective intervention. A key challenge in this task is the diverse and uncontrolled nature of medical environments, where procedures are often unscripted and highly variable. Numerous action classification benchmarks exist in the field, such as UCF101 [8], HMDB51 [9], Kinetics [10], Something-Something [11], and AVA [12]. However, the Trauma THOMPSON dataset stands out as the first egocentric video dataset specifically designed for medical procedure action recognition and anticipation, bringing unique value to the field.

2.3 Assessment Method

The performance of the proposed models for action recognition and action anticipation is evaluated using an automated, containerized pipeline to ensure reproducibility and objective benchmarking. The evaluation system aligns model predictions with ground truth annotations using temporal segments defined by start and end frame indices.

Evaluation Metrics. For each validated segment, the system assesses the model's ability to classify the ongoing activity (Recognition) and predict the immediate future activity (Anticipation). We define three primary metrics to quantify performance:

1. **Action Recognition Accuracy (Acc_{rec}):** Measures the proportion of correctly identified current actions over the total number of annotated segments.
2. **Action Anticipation Accuracy (Acc_{ant}):** Evaluates the model's foresight by calculating the ratio of correct next-action predictions to the total number of segments where a subsequent action is present.
3. **Final Accuracy (Acc_{final}):** An aggregate metric that represents the overall success rate across both tasks.

Mathematical Formulation. Let C_{rec} and C_{ant} denote the number of correct predictions for recognition and anticipation, respectively. Similarly, let N_{rec} and N_{ant} denote the total number of ground truth instances for each task. The metrics are computed as follows:

$$Acc_{rec} = \frac{C_{rec}}{N_{rec}}, \quad Acc_{ant} = \frac{C_{ant}}{N_{ant}} \tag{1}$$

The overall performance is captured by the Final Accuracy, which weights both tasks by their respective sample sizes:

$$Acc_{final} = \frac{C_{rec} + C_{ant}}{N_{rec} + N_{ant}} \tag{2}$$

This multi-task evaluation strategy ensures that models are rewarded for a comprehensive understanding of the procedural workflow, prioritizing both immediate situational awareness and predictive modeling.

3 Task 2: Emergency Procedure Hand Tracking

3.1 Datasets

Data Sources. For hand tracking, annotations were generated using a human-in-the-loop (HITL) framework combined with a bootstrapping strategy to ensure both scalability and accuracy. Initial preprocessing was performed using the MediaPipe hand detection model to automatically extract hand regions, including bounding box coordinates and corresponding spatial extents. These detections were further categorized as left or right hands based on a set of predefined heuristic rules. The resulting model-generated annotations served as preliminary labels, which were subsequently reviewed through human inspection. During this verification stage, annotators manually corrected errors such as misclassified hand laterality and inaccurately localized bounding boxes, thereby refining the quality and reliability of the final hand-tracking annotations.

Training and Test Case Characteristics. Each sample in the hand tracking dataset focuses on localizing hand movements and classifying hand laterality, as shown in Fig. 5. Annotations include precise bounding box coordinates, defined by $(x_{\min}, x_{\max}, y_{\min}, y_{\max})$, along with derived width and height values. In addition, each instance is labeled as either a left or right hand.

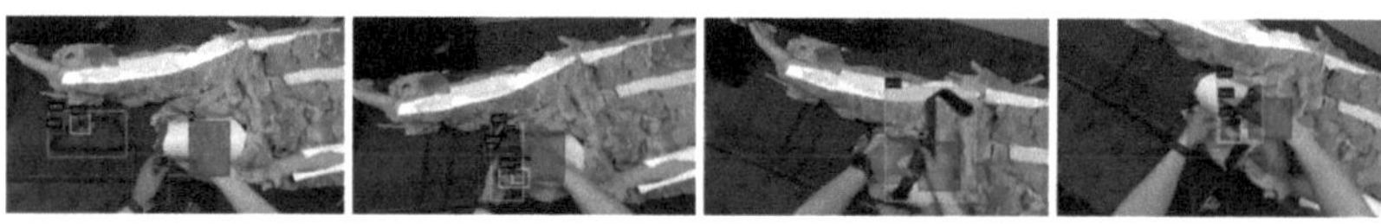

Fig. 5. Annotations of hands and objects.

The current training dataset consists of 30 videos comprising 65,127 annotated frames. For each frame, the annotations include: (i) bounding box coordinates, (ii) image dimensions, (iii) hand category (left or right), (iv) bounding box area, and (v) frame index. Ongoing annotation efforts are expanding the dataset, and at the time of challenge release, it is expected to include approximately 40 training videos with 104,392 instances (80%) and 10 testing videos with 26,098 instances (20%). This partitioning follows standard practices in machine learning, with flexibility for participants to further divide the training set into training and validation subsets.

Annotation Characteristics. Annotations adhere to the COCO format, where each detected hand is represented as an object instance with associated attributes. The evaluation protocol requires models to predict accurate bounding boxes in $(x, y, \text{width}, \text{height})$ format, along with the corresponding hand category label.

The annotation pipeline integrates automated detection with manual refinement. Initial hand localization is performed using the MediaPipe hand detection model to generate candidate bounding boxes [13]. These detections are subsequently assigned left/right labels based on heuristic rules. The resulting annotations are then reviewed by human annotators, who correct classification errors and adjust bounding box placements where necessary. Two annotators contributed to the creation and verification of the dataset.

To ensure consistency, bounding box coordinates are normalized, and frames without visible hands are excluded from the final dataset.

3.2 Assessment Aim

Hand tracking is a challenging but significant task. Such algorithm can assist care providers in identifying proper tools in a more straightforward manner. The task involves precisely capturing hand movements, classifying hand types (left or right hand), and recognizing medical tools in real-time. The ability to perform these tasks effectively is integral to enhancing decision-making in critical situations, and the presence of gloves makes these tasks even harder. The challenge focuses on advancing algorithms that can achieve high levels of accuracy and precision in detecting and tracking hands, even under the unpredictable conditions often encountered in medical environments. The performance of the task will largely improve the efficiency and quality of the surgeries. Additionally, it ensures the safety of patients, especially in urgent emergencies when patients meet the threaten of death.

3.3 Assessment Method: Hand Tracking

The assessment of hand tracking performance is conducted using an automated, containerized pipeline. Due to the specific architectural requirements of the Grand Challenge platform, bounding boxes are processed in a customized format rather than the standard COCO representation [14]. Specifically, boxes are defined by their vertex coordinates (corners), and frame association is handled through a string-based naming convention (e.g., *hand_side_frame_index*).

Spatial Localization Accuracy. Spatial accuracy is determined via the Intersection over Union (IoU) metric. Given a predicted box B_{pred} and a ground truth box B_{gt}, both defined by their corner vertices, we first extract the axis-aligned extrema:

$$x_{min} = \min(x_i), \quad x_{max} = \max(x_i), \quad y_{min} = \min(y_i), \quad y_{max} = \max(y_i) \quad (3)$$

The IoU is subsequently computed as:

$$IoU(B_{pred}, B_{gt}) = \frac{\text{Area}(B_{pred} \cap B_{gt})}{\text{Area}(B_{pred} \cup B_{gt})} \quad (4)$$

A prediction is considered valid if the IoU is ≥ 0.5.

Tracking Metrics and Aggregation. Temporal consistency and detection robustness are quantified using the Multiple Object Tracking Accuracy ($MOTA$) [15]. $MOTA$ accounts for False Positives (FP), False Negatives (FN), and Identity Switches ($IDSW$). The score for an individual hand class is formulated as:

$$MOTA = 1 - \frac{\sum_t (FN_t + FP_t + IDSW_t)}{\sum_t g_t} \quad (5)$$

where g_t represents the count of ground truth objects at frame t. As the task involves single-instance tracking per class (left/right hand), $IDSW$ is effectively nullified through consistent class labeling.

The final evaluation score ($MOTA_{avg}$) is the arithmetic mean of the individual hand scores:

$$MOTA_{avg} = \frac{MOTA_{left} + MOTA_{right}}{2} \tag{6}$$

This approach ensures that the evaluation captures the model's ability to maintain accurate tracks for both hands throughout the procedural sequence.

4 Task 3: Emergency Procedure Tool Detection

4.1 Datasets

Data Sources. For tool detection, annotations were generated using a semi-automated pipeline that combines pretrained detection models with human verification. Initial tool localization was performed using YOLOv11 [16], which produced candidate bounding boxes, spatial coordinates, and associated region attributes. These model-generated outputs were treated as provisional annotations and subsequently refined through a human-in-the-loop process. Annotators reviewed the detections to identify and correct errors, including misclassified tool categories and imprecise bounding box placements. This iterative refinement process improves annotation fidelity while maintaining scalability for large-scale dataset construction.

Training and Test Case Characteristics. In the tool detection task, each sample corresponds to a single image annotated with bounding boxes for medical instruments, where each instance represents a distinct detection and classification case, as shown in Fig. 5. The dataset comprises approximately 30,000 samples, with around 24,000 allocated for training and 6,000 for testing, following an 80/20 split consistent with standard machine learning practice. Participants may optionally partition the training set further to create a validation subset.

Annotation Characteristics. Annotations are provided in the YOLO format, where each object instance is encoded by its class label and normalized bounding box parameters ($x_{\text{center}}, y_{\text{center}}$, width, height), scaled relative to image dimensions [17]. Each bounding box is associated with a specific tool category, and evaluation requires accurate prediction of both localization and classification outputs. Three annotators contributed to the development and verification of the annotations.

The annotation workflow employs a semi-automated strategy. Pretrained YOLOv11 models were used to generate initial detections, including bounding box coordinates and tool category labels. These preliminary outputs were subsequently refined through manual review, during which annotators corrected misclassifications and adjusted bounding box placements. Annotation quality was further ensured through visual inspection, where bounding boxes and labels were overlaid on images for validation. Each image is associated with a single, finalized annotation set, eliminating ambiguity from multiple label sources.

To maintain dataset consistency, bounding box coordinates are normalized, and frames without relevant tool presence are excluded from the final dataset.

4.2 Assessment Aim

Emergency procedure tool detection is a fundamental yet critically important task in the Trauma Thompson Challenge. This type of algorithm is designed to detect crucial medical instruments throughout the entire emergency response process. Assisted by hand tracking, the algorithm aids healthcare providers in swiftly identifying every medical device involved in an emergency scenario, thereby enabling precise emergency support measures. Therefore, accurate identification of each emergency tool is of utmost importance. Operating under various unpredictable medical conditions, recognizing medical instruments that may differ in color, shape, but share the same function remains highly challenging. An accurate and broadly applicable emergency tool detection algorithm serves as the cornerstone for implementing emergency procedures, ensuring that the patient's emergency care process is conducted rapidly, correctly, and effectively.

4.3 Assessment Method

The evaluation of the surgical tool detection task is performed using a containerized pipeline on the Grand Challenge platform. This methodology accounts for specific platform requirements regarding data formats and metric aggregation to ensure clinical relevance and technical rigor.

Input and Output Formats. The assessment environment utilizes the .mha (MetaImage) format for medical video data, a departure from the common JPEG or PNG formats used during model development. Furthermore, predictions are rendered in Grand Challenge's customized vertex based bounding box JSON format. To utilize standard evaluation libraries, we transform these vertex coordinates (x_i, y_i) into COCO format, defined by the top left coordinate $(x_{\min}, y_{\min})$, width w, and height h, where $x_{\min} = \min(x_i)$, $y_{\min} = \min(y_i)$, $w = \max(x_i) - x_{\min}$, and $h = \max(y_i) - y_{\min}$.

Evaluation Metrics. Performance is quantified using the Mean Average Precision (mAP) across the COCO IoU thresholds $[0.5 : 0.05 : 0.95]$. The Intersection over Union (IoU), which determines the overlap between a prediction (B_p) and ground truth (B_{gt}), is calculated as:

$$IoU(B_p, B_{gt}) = \frac{\text{Area}(B_p \cap B_{gt})}{\text{Area}(B_p \cup B_{gt})} \tag{7}$$

For each tool category, the Average Precision (AP) is computed by calculating the area under the precision-recall curve:

$$AP = \int_0^1 p(r)\, dr \tag{8}$$

where $p(r)$ denotes precision as a function of recall r.

Global Aggregation. Given the varying tool density across different clinical cases, we employ a weighted average strategy to determine the final submission score (mAP_{final}). This ensures that sequences with a higher volume of ground truth annotations (N_i) exert a proportional influence on the total metric:

$$mAP_{final} = \frac{\sum_{i=1}^{n}(mAP_i \times N_i)}{\sum_{i=1}^{n} N_i} \tag{9}$$

where n is the total number of .mha files and mAP_i is the precision score for the i-th file.

5 Task 4: Realism Assessment

5.1 Datasets

Data Sources. The realism detection task utilizes the same egocentric procedure videos as those used in the action recognition and action anticipation tasks. These videos were captured using head-mounted cameras (GoPro Hero 7 or higher) in controlled environments designed to simulate realistic field conditions. The recordings provide high-resolution visual data suitable for evaluating perceptual realism.

Training and Test Case Characteristics. In the realism detection task, each sample consists of a procedural video paired with a corresponding realism score provided for both training and testing sets. The objective is to predict a scalar realism score for each video in the test set.

The dataset includes 177 videos, partitioned into 141 training samples (80%) and 36 testing samples (20%), following standard machine learning practice. Participants may optionally further divide the training set into training and validation subsets.

Annotation Characteristics. Realism is quantified on a scale from 0 to 10, based on a structured evaluation protocol. The score is derived from a set of predefined criteria capturing perceptual attributes such as motion characteristics, presence of injuries, depiction of bodily fluids, anatomical plausibility, and overall human likeness. Each criterion is assessed in a binary manner, and the final score is obtained by aggregating these responses.

Annotations were produced through systematic human evaluation, with two annotators independently reviewing the videos to ensure consistency and reliability. Each video is associated with a single finalized realism score, avoiding ambiguity from multiple annotations. The ground truth labels, along with corresponding video identifiers, are provided to participants in CSV format.

5.2 Assessment Aim

The realism assessment task requires participants to identify how realistic a simulated trauma procedure video appears from an egocentric point of view. Algorithms must be able to identify the realism of a video segment, using information about the procedure including steps, tools, and other important aspects of surgery. This would allow for the curation of higher quality training datasets, which would allow algorithms to learn the most accurate and realistic surgical processes, an essential step of improving accuracy in trauma care delivery assistance.

5.3 Assessment Method

The realism assessment task evaluates the model's ability to quantify the fidelity of simulated life-saving procedures. This task utilizes the same egocentric GoPro-recorded video dataset employed in the action recognition and anticipation tasks to ensure a holistic evaluation of the procedural sequences.

Scoring and Evaluation Pipeline. Models are required to assign a realism score, $s \in [0, 10]$, to each video sequence. A score of 0 represents a complete lack of procedural realism, while a score of 10 denotes an expert-level, highly realistic execution. The evaluation is performed within a containerized environment where model predictions are matched against expert-provided ground truth scores via a standardized mapping.

Performance Metrics. To measure the accuracy of the predicted scores, we employ Mean Squared Error (MSE) and Root Mean Squared Error ($RMSE$). Let n be the total number of evaluation cases, y_i be the ground truth score for video i, and $\hat{y}_i$ be the model's predicted score.

The MSE represents the average squared deviation of the predictions from the ground truth:

$$MSE = \frac{1}{n}\sum_{i=1}^{n}(y_i - \hat{y}_i)^2 \tag{10}$$

The primary metric for ranking and performance comparison is the $RMSE$, calculated as:

$$RMSE = \sqrt{\frac{1}{n}\sum_{i=1}^{n}(y_i - \hat{y}_i)^2} \tag{11}$$

The $RMSE$ serves as a representative measure of the average error magnitude, expressed in the same units as the 0–10 realism scale, thereby providing an intuitive assessment of the model's predictive precision relative to expert judgment.

6 Task 5: Visual Question Answering

6.1 Datasets

Data Sources. VQA task leverages the same egocentric procedure videos used in the other tasks. Annotations are entirely human-generated, with experienced annotators constructing question–answer pairs grounded in the visual and procedural context of the recordings. To improve annotation efficiency and consistency, answers were propagated across frames exhibiting similar visual content. The dataset is derived from recordings performed by trained medical professionals, ensuring that the generated questions and answers reflect realistic procedural scenarios.

Training and Test Case Characteristics. For the VQA task, images are extracted from procedural videos and annotated with multiple question–answer pairs per image. Each question is associated with at least one concise answer, and the training annotations are publicly available, while the test set provides only questions for evaluation. The dataset comprises approximately 594,000 instances, with around 475,000 samples (80%) for training and 119,000 samples (20%) for testing, following standard data partitioning practices.

Annotation Characteristics. All annotations are human-generated to ensure contextual accuracy, with annotators formulating questions and answers that emphasize procedural understanding, tool usage, and decision-making. The annotation process was conducted and reviewed by three annotators, ensuring consistency and quality. Each image is associated with a single, finalized set of annotations, eliminating ambiguity from multiple label sources.

6.2 Assessment Aim

The VQA task requires participants to answer various questions about egocentric images from surgical procedures. They must be able to identify the correct answers to any given question relating to tools, next steps, and other components of surgery. Although multiple VQA datasets exist (VQAv2, Coco, etc.) [14,18], the Trauma THOMPSON VQA dataset is unique as it is the first to utilize egocentric trauma surgery data when prompting the participant for an answer. The algorithms implemented by participants must be innovative enough to analyze complex trauma surgery images and be able to generate an answer to any question related to that image. This aids in more accurate decision-making and less confusion among healthcare providers performing trauma care procedures.

6.3 Assessment Method

The Visual Question Answering (VQA) task is assessed through a dual-metric framework that balances strict correctness with semantic similarity. Model performance is primarily quantified using Exact-Match Accuracy, defined as:

$$Acc = \frac{1}{N}\sum_{i=1}^{N} \mathbb{1}(\hat{y}_i = y_i) \tag{12}$$

where N denotes the total number of test samples, $\hat{y}_i$ represents the predicted answer, y_i is the ground truth reference, and $\mathbb{1}(\cdot)$ is an indicator function for exact string matching.

To account for lexical overlap and provide a finer differentiation of performance, the BLEU score is utilized as a secondary metric. The evaluation protocol follows a hierarchical ranking strategy: participants are first ranked by Accuracy, with the BLEU score serving as the tie-breaking criterion for identical Accuracy results. In accordance with standard evaluation practices, missing predictions are treated as incorrect and assigned a score of zero, thereby ensuring that the final rankings reflect both the accuracy and the completeness of the submissions.

7 Assessment Methodologies and Technical Constraints

The evaluation for all challenge tasks was conducted via a containerized environment on the Grand Challenge platform, ensuring a standardized and reproducible benchmarking process. While the challenge provided high-quality expert annotations, the platform imposed specific infrastructure requirements that diverged from common computer vision workflows.

For image-centric tasks, including Object Detection (Task 3) and Visual Question Answering (Task 5), the platform required the use of the .mha file format for input data. Although standard in certain medical imaging domains, this choice is unconventional for typical object detection and VQA pipelines, which primarily utilize JPEG or PNG formats. Furthermore, the platform required predictions to be rendered in a customized vertex-based JSON format rather than standard COCO or YOLO schemas. These technical barriers necessitated the development of complex transformation layers to convert standard model outputs into platform-compliant formats, potentially increasing the entry threshold for participants in these specific categories.

8 Methods and Results

This section details the outcomes of the Trauma THOMPSON Challenge 2025 for the three tasks that received active participant submissions: Action Recognition and Anticipation (Task 1), Hand Tracking (Task 2), and Realism Assessment (Task 4). Task 3 (Object Detection) and Task 5 (Visual Question Answering) did not receive any submissions. As previously noted, a primary factor for the lack of participation in these tasks may be attributed to the requirement of the .mha file format on the Grand Challenge platform, which is not a conventional standard for the broader object detection and VQA research communities.

8.1 Challenge Participation

The Trauma THOMPSON Challenge 2025 received broad interest from the medical computer vision and surgical AI communities on the Grand Challenge platform. In total, 11 teams comprising 23 formally registered team members were formed, and 6 teams submitted algorithms for evaluation. The participating teams represented diverse university-based research groups across computer vision, biomedical engineering, medical AI, and surgical data science, highlighting the interdisciplinary academic relevance of egocentric trauma procedure understanding and AI-assisted emergency care.

8.2 Task 1: Action Recognition and Anticipation

The action recognition and anticipation task was evaluated based on a unified accuracy metric representing the ratio of correct estimates for both current and subsequent actions. The leaderboard is shown in Table 1. Performance was led by team **NCT-TSO**, which achieved a top score of 0.6148. Their methodology utilized a 3D convolutional neural network (X3D-M) for spatiotemporal feature extraction, augmented with a unidirectional LSTM to model the temporal evolution of procedural segments. In contrast, team **Lind** placed second with a score of 0.3061 using an adapted DINOv2 foundation model. A significant challenge across submissions was the introduction of JIT procedures in the test set.

8.3 Task 2: Hand Tracking

Hand tracking performance was quantified using MOTA and the leaderboard is shown in Table 1. Team **MediSC_Godhand** secured the first position with a score of 0.5088. Team **BIOMED** followed in second place with a score of 0.3417, utilizing a YOLOv8-L architecture. Their findings emphasized that a data-centric workflow yielded higher performance gains than fundamental architectural changes, including extensive exploratory data analysis and optimized input resolutions (832×832). Team **KDSUN** achieved third place with a score of 0.3330 using a YOLOv10-based multi-task framework. While team KDSUN demonstrated effective laterality classification (67% left hand, 71% right hand), they noted that distinguishing hands from complex surgical backgrounds remains a persistent challenge, with nearly half of hand instances being confused with the background.

8.4 Task 4: Realism Assessment

The realism assessment task required participants to estimate a score between 0 and 10. Team **NCT-TSO** provided the only submission for this task, achieving a RMSE of 0.7854. Their approach employed a spatiotemporal X3D-M feature extractor with a dedicated regression head to evaluate holistic video representations against expert-assigned ground truth scores.

Table 1. Leaderboard Results for the Trauma THOMPSON Challenge 2025.

Task	Metric	Team (Algorithm)	Score
Task 1	Accuracy	NCT-TSO (Actions)	0.6148
		Lind (DINOv2)	0.3061
Task 2	MOTA	MediSC_Godhand (GodHand)	0.5088
		BIOMED (YOLOv8-L)	0.3417
		KDSUN (YOLOv10)	0.3330
Task 4	RMSE	NCT-TSO (Realism)	0.7854

9 Discussion

The outcomes of the Trauma THOMPSON Challenge 2025 demonstrate a remarkable leap in the maturity of procedural understanding compared to the 2023 results. In the initial challenge, the best-performing action recognition models—leveraging SlowFast and VideoSwin architectures—achieved a top-1 accuracy of approximately 35.27%. In contrast, the 2025 leaderboard shows that team NCT-TSO nearly doubled this performance, reaching an accuracy of 61.48% through a sophisticated hybrid CNN-LSTM framework. This improvement highlights a shift from basic spatiotemporal feature extraction to more holistic procedural modeling. Furthermore, while the 2023 challenge noted that action anticipation was significantly more difficult, yielding a top-1 accuracy of only 23.67%, the 2025 participants demonstrated far greater predictive robustness, even when faced with the increased variability of the test set.

An important advancement in the 2025 challenge is the proactive addressing of the "domain disparity" between manikin-based simulators and real patients, which was explicitly cited as a core limitation in the 2023 findings. By introducing Task 4 (Realism Assessment), the 2025 challenge provides a formal mechanism for quantifying clinical fidelity, a step that allows for more effective training on simulated data while preparing models for real-patient contexts. Additionally, the transition from standard CNN-based backbones used in 2023 to the evaluation of large-scale foundation models like DINOv2 and ActionCLIP in 2025 demonstrates the challenge's commitment to cutting-edge AI research. These foundation models provide the few-shot capabilities necessary to handle the long-tailed class distribution that remains a characteristic of realistic medical procedure datasets.

The successful expansion of the task scope to include hand tracking and JIT procedures further elevates the challenge's relevance to operational medicine.

While 2023 focused on four primary tasks within a satellite event framework, the 2025 challenge successfully integrated more nuanced tasks like hand laterality classification and the recognition of improvised tools. Although the JIT scenarios introduced a performance gap, their inclusion is a testament to the challenge's rigorous commitment to real-world unpredictability, ensuring that models are tested not just on standardized workflows but also on the adaptive logic required in humanitarian crises and battlefield medicine.

10 Conclusion

The Trauma THOMPSON Challenge 2025 has established itself as a premier benchmark for emergency procedure video understanding, showing extraordinary growth since its inception in 2023. The nearly twofold increase in action recognition accuracy and the successful deployment of multi-task tracking and realism assessment frameworks demonstrate the great potential for AI-guided trauma care. By addressing the technical and domain-specific hurdles identified in earlier iterations, this challenge has provided a clear roadmap for developing robust and autonomous decision-support systems. The insights gained from the participants' methodologies offer promising evidence that AI can successfully navigate the complexities of life-saving interventions in resource-limited settings. Ultimately, the 2025 challenge stands as a significant contribution to the goal of improving survival outcomes in austere environments through innovative, reliable, and clinically grounded artificial intelligence.

References

1. Wachs, J.P., Kirkpatrick, A.W., Tisherman, S.A.: Procedural telementoring in rural, underdeveloped, and austere settings: origins, present challenges, and future perspectives. Annu. Rev. Biomed. Eng. **23**(1), 115–139 (2021). https://doi.org/10.1146/annurev-bioeng-083120-023315
2. Shackelford, S.A., et al.: Case-control analysis of prehospital death and prolonged field care survival during recent US military combat operations. J. Trauma Acute Care Surg. **91**(2), S186–S193 (2021). https://doi.org/10.1097/TA.0000000000003252
3. Riesberg, J., Powell, D., Loos, P.: The loss of the golden hour. Spec. Warfare Mag **30**(1), 49–51 (2017)
4. Bhattarai, H.K., Bhusal, S., Barone-Adesi, F., Hubloue, I.: Prehospital emergency care in low- and middle-income countries: a systematic review. Prehosp. Disaster Med. **38**(4), 495–512 (2023). https://doi.org/10.1017/S1049023X23006088
5. Zhuo, Y., et al.: Overview of the Trauma THOMPSON challenge at MICCAI 2023. In: Bao, R., Grant, E., Kirkpatrick, A., Wachs, J., Ou, Y. (eds.) AI for Brain Lesion Detection and Trauma Video Action Recognition, pp. 47–60. Springer, Cham (2025). https://doi.org/10.1007/978-3-031-71626-3_7
6. Zhuo, Y., et al.: An egocentric life-saving interventional procedure dataset of actions, medical questions. maneuvers and tools. Sci. Data **13**(1), 51 (2025). https://doi.org/10.1038/s41597-025-06365-y

7. Damen, D., et al.: The EPIC-KITCHENS Dataset: collection, Challenges and Baselines (2020). arXiv:2005.00343 [cs]
8. Soomro, K., Zamir, A.R., Shah, M.: UCF101: a dataset of 101 human actions classes from videos in the wild. ArXiv abs/1212.0402 (2012). https://doi.org/10.48550/ARXIV.1212.0402
9. Kuehne, H., Jhuang, H., Garrote, E., Poggio, T., Serre, T.: HMDB: a large video database for human motion recognition. In: 2011 International Conference on Computer Vision, pp. 2556–2563. IEEE, Barcelona (2011). https://doi.org/10.1109/ICCV.2011.6126543
10. Kay, W., et al.: The kinetics human action video dataset. CoRR abs/1705.06950 (2017). arXiv:1705.06950
11. Goyal, R., et al.: The "something something" video database for learning and evaluating visual common sense. In: Proceedings of the IEEE International Conference on Computer Vision (2017). https://doi.org/10.48550/ARXIV.1706.04261
12. Gu, C., et al.: AVA: a video dataset of spatio-temporally localized atomic visual actions. In: 2018 IEEE/CVF Conference on Computer Vision and Pattern Recognition, pp. 6047–6056 (2018). https://doi.org/10.1109/CVPR.2018.00633
13. Lugaresi, C., et al.: MediaPipe: a framework for building perception pipelines (2019). arXiv:1906.08172 [cs]
14. Lin, T.-Y., et al.: Microsoft COCO: common objects in context (2014). https://doi.org/10.48550/ARXIV.1405.0312. Version Number: 3
15. Hassan, S., Mujtaba, G., Rajput, A., Fatima, N.: Multi-object tracking: a systematic literature review. Multimed. Tools Appl. **83**(14), 43439–43492 (2023). https://doi.org/10.1007/s11042-023-17297-3
16. Khanam, R., Hussain, M.: YOLOv11: an overview of the key architectural enhancements (2024). https://doi.org/10.48550/arXiv.2410.17725, arXiv:2410.17725 [cs]
17. Redmon, J., Divvala, S., Girshick, R., Farhadi, A.: You only look once: unified, real-time object detection (2015). https://doi.org/10.48550/ARXIV.1506.02640. Version Number: 5
18. Agrawal, A., et al.: VQA: visual question answering (2016). arXiv:1505.00468 [cs]

NCT-TSO Submission to The Trauma THOMPSON Challenge 2025

Isabel Funke[1,2](✉), Hanna Hoffmann[1], and Stefanie Speidel[1,2]

[1] Department of Translational Surgical Oncology, National Center for Tumor Diseases (NCT), NCT/UCC Dresden, a partnership between DKFZ, Faculty of Medicine and University Hospital Carl Gustav Carus, TUD Dresden University of Technology, and Helmholtz-Zentrum Dresden- Rossendorf (HZDR), Dresden, Germany

Isabel.Funke@nct-dresden.de

[2] The Centre for Tactile Internet with Human-in-the-Loop (CeTI), TUD Dresden University of Technology, Dresden, Germany

Abstract. The Trauma THOMPSON Challenge 2025 aims to unlock the potential of artificial intelligence to provide real-time decision support to remote frontline providers during lifesaving medical procedures. To facilitate research in this domain, the challenge offers a dataset of egocentric videos captured with head-mounted cameras, documenting simulated emergency care procedures performed on realistic manikins. Further, the challenge designs five clinically relevant video understanding and visual recognition tasks. In this report, we present our submissions to task 1 (action recognition and anticipation) and task 4 (realism assessment). Our methods build on a 3D convolutional neural network for spatiotemporal video modeling, augmented with a recurrent neural network to capture the temporal evolution of medical actions in task 1. On the unseen challenge test set, the submitted solutions achieve an overall accuracy of 61.5 % in the action recognition and anticipation task and a root mean squared error of 0.785 in the realism assessment task.

Keywords: Emergency care · Medical simulation · Video understanding · Action recognition · Action anticipation · Realism assessment

1 Introduction

The Trauma THOMPSON Challenge 2025 aims to explore AI-based real-time guidance to frontline providers during high-stakes and lifesaving procedures. To study how well AI models can recognize medical actions, anticipate next steps, detect tools, track hand motion, or answer clinical questions, the challenge provides a dataset of egocentric videos, acquired using head-mounted cameras. These videos record simulated emergency care procedures that are performed on various medical simulators by military medics and medical experts.

J. P. Wachs et al. (Eds.): TrackRAD/TTC 2025, LNCS 16474, pp. 92–100, 2027.
https://doi.org/10.1007/978-3-032-35046-6_9

In this report, we describe our submissions to challenge task 1 (action recognition and action anticipation) and challenge task 4 (realism assessment). Our solutions are based on the established X3D convolutional neural network [4] for spatiotemporal video modeling.

Table 1. Egocentric video dataset provided for tasks 1 and 4

Type	Procedure	video count	mean duration
P01	Tracheostomy	29	80.9 s
P02	Tube thoracostomy	27	118.7 s
P03	Intraosseous insertion	24	51.8 s
P04	Needle thoracostomy	30	45.3 s
P05	Tourniquet application	31	42.1 s

The released challenge training data comprises a total of 141 videos of five different emergency care procedures: intraosseous insertion, needle thoracostomy, tourniquet application, tracheostomy, and tube thoracostomy. Table 1 shows the number of video recordings per procedure type as well as their average duration. An extended version of the dataset with 220 videos has been released recently [14].

With an average duration of less than two minutes, the recorded videos are of manageable length. Yet, video models like X3D are designed to model short video clips. Therefore, we break videos down into short snippets for analysis. In this report, a video snippet consists of 16 consecutive frames, which are extracted with a temporal resolution of 10 fps. This means that each snippet corresponds to 1.6 s of video. The spatial resolution of each frame in a snippet is 384 × 224 pixels. Figure 1 illustrates the concept.

We use the PyTorch [11] framework to implement our models and train models on a Nvidia RTX A5000 GPU with 24 GB of video RAM. The X3D model is initialized with the weights obtained after pretraining on the Kinetics dataset [2].

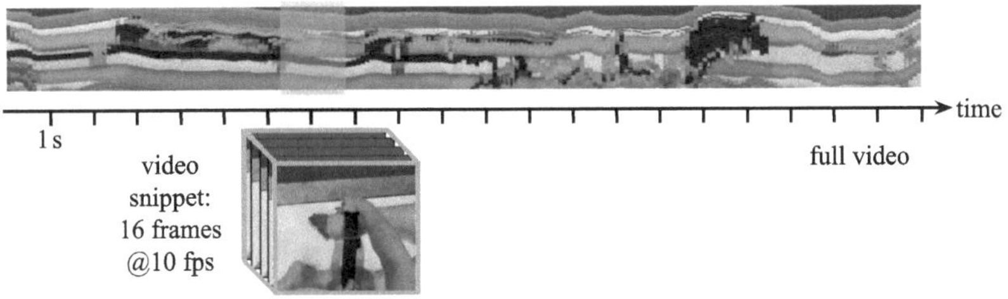

Fig. 1. Visualization of a video recording of a simulated tourniquet application. To illustrate the process along the temporal dimension, we show a videogram [3], where each video frame is reduced to a strip around its center column. 16 consecutive frames, highlighted in green, constitute a video snippet.

2 Submission to Task 1: Action Recognition and Action Anticipation

For task 1 of the Trauma THOMPSON Challenge 2025, a segmentation of each video is given, indicating the start and end times of atomic action segments. The task is to automatically recognize the action that is performed in each segment and to simultaneously anticipate the action that will be performed in the subsequent segment. Here, an action is defined as a pair of verb and noun, such as "identify wound", "position tourniquet", or "tighten strap".

The released challenge training data comprises 42 verb classes and 42 noun classes, which form 124 known verb-noun combinations. We summarize consecutive segments that are labeled as the same action as one long segment, which yields 2444 individual video segments in the training data.

The proposed evaluation metric for this task is overall accuracy, which is the ratio of correct estimates considering both the current and the next action. Given the challenge test set of videos V, we denote the sequence of ground truth actions in this video as $(a_{v,i})_{i=1}^{n_v}$, where n_v refers to the number of segments in video v. For $1 \leq i \leq n_v$, a solution to task 1 estimates the current action $\hat{a}_{v,i}$ and, if $i < n_v$, the next action $\hat{a}^+_{v,i}$ for the i-th segment in video v. Hence, the overall accuracy is computed as

$$\frac{\sum_{v \in V} |\{\hat{a}_{v,i} = a_{v,i} : 1 \leq i \leq n_v\}| + \sum_{v \in V} |\{\hat{a}^+_{v,i} = a_{v,i+1} : 1 \leq i \leq n_v - 1\}|}{\sum_{v \in V} n_v + \sum_{v \in V} (n_v - 1)} . \quad (1)$$

Notably, the challenge test set also includes just-in-time procedures, where improvised tools, such as belts, screwdrivers, and clothing, are used to perform life-saving interventions. Yet, no examples of just-in-time procedures were released as part of the training set. Therefore, we did not aim to explicitly design a solution that can generalize to video recordings of this kind.

2.1 Model Architecture

Our proposed solution for task 1 is presented in Fig. 2. Given a test video with action segment boundaries, we use a 3D CNN (X3D-M [4]) to compute a spatiotemporal feature representation of each video segment. Here, we divide long video segments into short snippets, which overlap slightly, and use the 3D CNN to compute spatiotemporal feature representations on each snippet individually. Then, the snippet-wise feature vectors are aggregated into a segment-level feature vector using global average pooling. In contrast, if a video segment is shorter than 1.6 s, we duplicate video frames at the beginning and at the end of the segment to obtain a 16-frame snippet.

Given a representation for each video segment, we apply a recurrent neural network (unidirectional LSTM [5]) to the sequence of segment features that represent one video. The LSTM consists of one layer and has 96 hidden units.

Using an LSTM on top helps to keep track of previously occurred action segments and to relate previous information to the current segment representation,

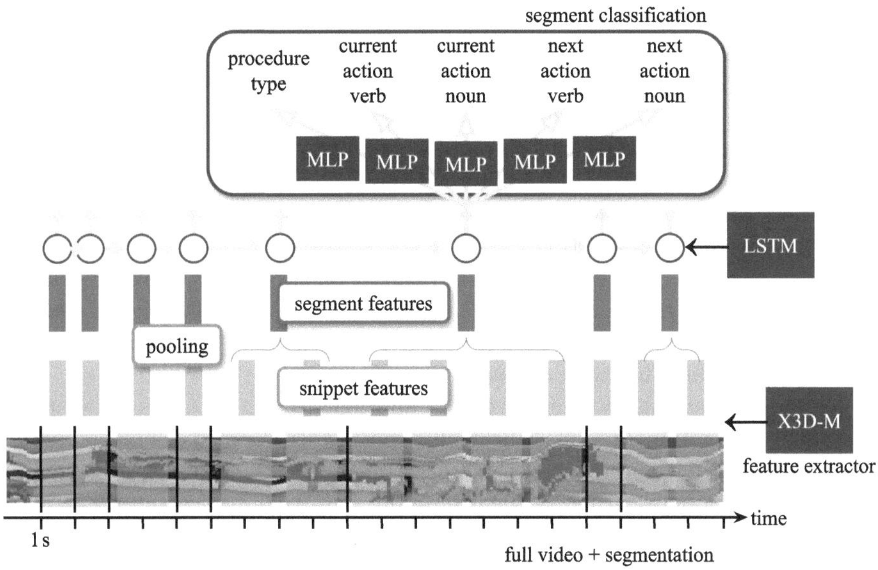

Fig. 2. NCT-TSO Submission to Task 1: We use a 3D CNN (X3D-M) to compute a spatiotemporal feature representation for each video segment and add a recurrent neural network (LSTM) to relate information from previous segments to the current one. On top of the LSTM, five classification heads (MLPs) estimate the current action verb and noun, the next action verb and noun, and the procedure type for each segment.

which is beneficial to estimate the current and the next action. Especially for action anticipation, we think that it is necessary to know what happened before in order to infer what could happen next.

To obtain the current and next action for each segment, we add 2-layer MLPs as classification heads. Based on the LSTM's cell state, the MLPs independently estimate the current action verb, the current action noun, the next action verb, the next action noun, and additionally the procedure type. With this approach, action verb and action noun are computed separately from each other, which could help with generalization to previously unseen verb-noun combinations.

Notably, the X3D feature extractor is trained independently of the LSTM and the classification heads, which is detailed in the following.

2.2 Model Training

Step 1: Training the 3D CNN for Visual Feature Extraction. To learn meaningful snippet and segment features, we first train the 3D CNN on isolated video segments to recognize only the current action and the procedure type. Here, we temporarily add three MLPs as classification heads to estimate the procedure type, the current action verb, and the current action noun based on the segment feature, which – as explained before – is obtained by pooling over individual snippet features computed by the 3D CNN.

In contrast to inference time, where snippets are extracted from long video segments at equal distances and with overlap, snippets are sampled randomized and sparsely at training time. The number of snippets is chosen such that they cover about 65 % of the frames in the segment. To represent all parts of a segment, the segment is divided into uniform partitions and from within each of them, one snippet is sampled [13].

To augment the data, we use the Albumentations library [1] to apply stochastic transformations to the video frames, including color transformations, geometric transformations, and horizontal flipping. The same transformation is applied to all frames within the same snippet.

For model training, we minimize the unweighted sum of the cross-entropy losses on each of the three classification tasks (procedure type, current action verb, current action noun) using the Adam optimizer [7]. The model is trained for up to 1000 epochs, using gradient clipping [10] with a maximum norm of 1 and a learning rate schedule that linearly increases the learning rate up to a maximum value of $3 \cdot 10^{-5}$ during a warm-up period of 333 epochs and switches to cosine decay afterwards to smoothly decrease the learning rate until the end of training [9]. Here, we keep the model that achieves highest action recognition accuracy on the validation data, which is a quarter of the challenge training data that we hold out.

Step 2: Training the LSTM on Frozen Segment Features. With the 3D CNN trained and frozen, we train the LSTM and the classification heads on sequences of segment features, where each sequence represents the consecutive segments in one video. To reduce overfitting, we apply dropout [12] (dropout probability $p = 0.5$) to the segment features.

We minimize the unweighted sum of the cross-entropy losses, aggregated over all segments in a video, on each of the five classification tasks (procedure type, current action verb, current action noun, next action verb, next action noun) using the Adam optimizer [7]. The model is trained for up to 1000 epochs using gradient clipping [10] (maximum norm = 1) and an initial learning rate of 10^{-3}, which is smoothly decreased using cosine decay [9]. We keep the model that achieves highest overall accuracy (see Eq. (1)) on the validation data.

2.3 Challenge Submission

To compete in the challenge, we create a simple model ensemble using the following strategy: We randomly split the released training data into four folds of similar size, with stratification based on the procedure type. Then, we train four 3D CNN-LSTM models on different subsets of the training data, following a cross-validation scheme. This means that we use the i-th fold as validation data and the remaining folds as training data to train the i-th model ($1 \leq i \leq 4$).

To estimate the sequences of current and next actions on a test video, we apply each of the 3D CNN-LSTM models to the video and average their outputs, in particular the logits after softmax. This approach achieves an overall accuracy of 0.615 on the challenge test set.

3 Submission to Task 4: Realism Assessment

For task 4 of the Trauma THOMPSON Challenge 2025, a video is given and the video's realism, compared to real-world medical scenarios, is to be assessed. More specifically, a realism score between 0 and 10 needs to be estimated.

Here, the true realism score is defined as the number of satisfied criteria. A total of ten criteria are predefined. They cover aspects of the patient's condition, including movement, presence of injuries, bodily fluids, anatomical coherence, and overall human-like appearance.

Besides the 141 videos from task 1, five additional videos were released for task 4, one for each procedure type. These additional videos involve human patients and thus have higher realism scores assigned.

The proposed evaluation metric for this task is the root mean squared error (RMSE). Given the challenge test set V, where r_v denotes the ground truth realism score for video $v \in V$ and $\hat{r}_v$ denotes the estimated realism score, RMSE is computed as

$$\sqrt{\frac{1}{|V|} \sum_{v \in V} (\hat{r}_v - r_v)^2} \,. \tag{2}$$

3.1 Model Architecture

Our proposed solution for task 4 is presented in Fig. 3. First, we divide the test video into short overlapping video snippets. Then, we use a 3D CNN (X3D-M [4]) to compute a spatiotemporal feature representation of each of the snippets. To obtain a holistic video representation, we aggregate the snippet-wise feature vectors into a video-level feature vector using global average pooling. Given the video feature, a 2-layer MLP is employed as regression head to estimate the realism score. An additional 2-layer MLP is employed as classification head to recognize the procedure type.

3.2 Model Training

We train the complete architecture end to end on full videos. Here, we minimize the sum of two losses: cross-entropy loss on the procedure type recognition task and Huber loss ($\delta = 0.5$) [6] on the realism score regression task. We weight the Huber loss for realism assessment by a factor of 4 compared to the cross-entropy loss for procedure type recognition.

In contrast to inference time, where snippets are extracted at equal distances and with overlap, we randomly sample snippet positions at training time so that the extracted snippets cover about 75 % of all frames in the video. To consider all parts of the video, the video v is first divided uniformly into n_v segments and then one snippet is extracted at a random position from within each segment [13].

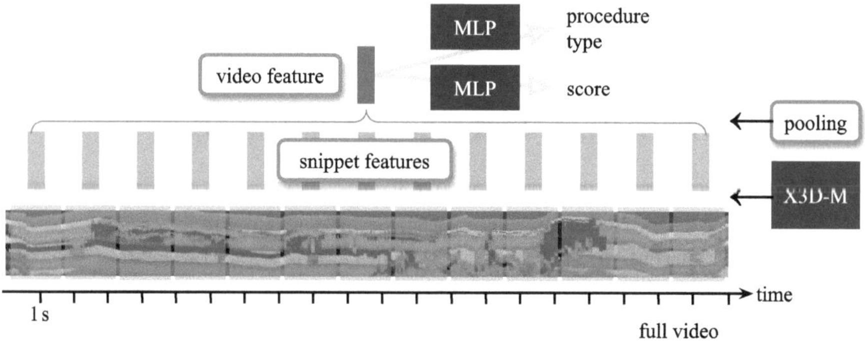

Fig. 3. NCT-TSO Submission to Task 4: We use a 3D CNN (X3D-M) to compute a holistic spatiotemporal feature representation for the video, based on which two MLPs estimate the realism score and the procedure type.

To augment the data, we use the Albumentations library [1] to apply stochastic transformations to the video frames, including color transformations, geometric transformations, and horizontal flipping. The same transformation is applied to all frames within the same snippet.

We train the model for up to 450 epochs, using the Adam optimizer [7] with gradient clipping [10] (maximum norm = 1) and an initial learning rate of 10^{-4}, which is smoothly decreased during training using cosine decay [9]. The batch size is one video or n_v video snippets. On long videos, which correspond to more than 14 snippets ($n_v > 14$), we aggregate gradients for the 3D CNN feature extractor sequentially over smaller micro-batches [8].

We keep the model that achieves lowest RMSE (see Eq. (2)) on the validation data, which is a quarter of the challenge training data that we hold out.

3.3 Challenge Submission

To compete in the challenge, we create a simple model ensemble using the following strategy: We randomly split the released training data (except for the five additional real videos) into four folds of similar size, with stratification based on the procedure type. Here, we aim to distribute videos with low and high realism scores equally between folds. Then, we train four models on different subsets of the training data, following a cross-validation scheme. Here, we use the i-th fold as validation data and the remaining folds plus the five real videos as training data to train the i-th model ($1 \leq i \leq 4$).

To obtain the realism score of a test video, we apply each model to the video and average the scores that they compute. This approach achieves a root mean squared error of 0.785 on the challenge test set.

4 Conclusion

The evaluation results demonstrate the potential of simple deep learning architectures, based on an established efficient spatiotemporal convolutional model (X3D), for medical video understanding. In both task 1 and task 4, our solutions rank first on the challenge's 2025 leaderbord, providing an important baseline for future work in this domain. Still, there is room for improvement, especially on the action recognition and anticipation task. More annotated training data seems to be required.

Acknowledgments. Funded by the German Research Foundation (DFG, Deutsche Forschungsgemeinschaft) as part of Germany's Excellence Strategy EXC 2050/1 Project ID 390696704 Cluster of Excellence "Centre for Tactile Internet with Human-in-the-Loop" (CeTI) of Technische Universität Dresden.

Supported by the project "Next Generation AI Computing (gAIn)," funded by the Bavarian Ministry of Science and the Arts and the Saxon Ministry for Science, Culture, and Tourism.

Disclosure of Interests. The authors have no competing interests to declare that are relevant to the content of this article.

References

1. Buslaev, A., Iglovikov, V.I., Khvedchenya, E., Parinov, A., Druzhinin, M., Kalinin, A.A.: Albumentations: fast and flexible image augmentations. Information **11**(2), 125 (2020). https://doi.org/10.3390/info11020125. version 1.4.4
2. Carreira, J., Zisserman, A.: Quo vadis, action recognition? A new model and the Kinetics dataset. In: IEEE Conference on Computer Vision and Pattern Recognition (CVPR), pp. 4724–4733 (2017). https://doi.org/10.1109/CVPR.2017.502
3. Davis, M.: Media streams: an iconic visual language for video representation. In: Baecker, R.M., Grudin, J., Buxton, W., Greenberg, S. (eds.) Readings in Human-Computer Interaction: Toward the Year 2000, 2 edn., pp. 854–866. Interactive Technologies, Morgan Kaufmann (1995). https://doi.org/10.1016/B978-0-08-051574-8.50089-3
4. Feichtenhofer, C.: X3D: expanding architectures for efficient video recognition. In: IEEE/CVF Conference on Computer Vision and Pattern Recognition (CVPR), pp. 200–210 (2020). https://doi.org/10.1109/CVPR42600.2020.00028
5. Hochreiter, S., Schmidhuber, J.: Long short-term memory. Neural Comput. **9**(8), 1735–1780 (1997). https://doi.org/10.1162/neco.1997.9.8.1735
6. Huber, P.J.: Robust estimation of a location parameter. Ann. Math. Stat. **35**(1), 73–101 (1964). https://doi.org/10.1214/aoms/1177703732
7. Kingma, D.P., Ba, J.: Adam: a method for stochastic optimization. In: International Conference for Learning Representations (ICLR) (2015). https://doi.org/10.48550/arXiv.1412.6980
8. Liu, S., Xu, M., Zhao, C., Zhao, X., Ghanem, B.: ETAD: training action detection end to end on a laptop. In: IEEE/CVF Conference on Computer Vision and Pattern Recognition Workshops (CVPRW), pp. 4525–4534 (2023). https://doi.org/10.1109/CVPRW59228.2023.00476

9. Loshchilov, I., Hutter, F.: SGDR: stochastic gradient descent with warm restarts. In: International Conference on Learning Representations (ICLR) (2017). https://openreview.net/forum?id=Skq89Scxx
10. Pascanu, R., Mikolov, T., Bengio, Y.: On the difficulty of training recurrent neural networks. In: International Conference on Machine Learning (ICML). Proceedings of Machine Learning Research, vol. 28, pp. 1310–1318 (2013). http://proceedings.mlr.press/v28/pascanu13.html
11. Paszke, A., et al.: PyTorch: an imperative style, high-performance deep learning library. In: Advances in Neural Information Processing Systems, vol. 32 (2019). https://proceedings.neurips.cc/paper/2019/hash/bdbca288fee7f92f2bfa9f7012727740-Abstract.html
12. Srivastava, N., Hinton, G., Krizhevsky, A., Sutskever, I., Salakhutdinov, R.: Dropout: a simple way to prevent neural networks from overfitting. J. Mach. Learn. Res. **15**(56), 1929–1958 (2014). http://jmlr.org/papers/v15/srivastava14a.html
13. Wang, L., et al.: Temporal segment networks: towards good practices for deep action recognition. In: Leibe, B., Matas, J., Sebe, N., Welling, M. (eds.) ECCV 2016. LNCS, vol. 9912, pp. 20–36. Springer, Cham (2016). https://doi.org/10.1007/978-3-319-46484-8_2
14. Zhuo, Y., et al.: An egocentric life-saving interventional procedure dataset of actions, medical questions, maneuvers and tools. Sci. Data **13**(51) (2025). https://doi.org/10.1038/s41597-025-06365-y

A Data-Driven Workflow for Real-Time Hand Tracking in Surgical Video

Konstantinos Georgas(✉), Theodoros P. Vagenas, and George K. Matsopoulos

Biomedical Engineering Lab (BEL), School of Electrical and Computer Engineering, National Technical University of Athens, 15780 Athens, Greece
{kostasgeo,tpvagenas,gmatsopoulos}@biomed.ntua.gr
https://www.biomed.ntua.gr/

Abstract. Accurate and real-time observation of the surgeon's hands in real time is a fundamental component in the development of computer-assisted surgical procedures. However, challenges such as instrument occlusion, motion blur and the use of surgical gloves require effective and specialized solutions. This study presents the methodology behind the second-placed solution for Task 2 of the Trauma THOMPSON Challenge 2025. The approach is defined by a comprehensive data-driven workflow that begins with extensive Exploratory Data Analysis (EDA) to understand the unique characteristics of the available data. The results of the analysis directly informed the development of a customized data pre-processing pipeline, as well as the tuning of hyperparameters for an object detection method based on YOLOv8. By systematically addressing issues of redundancy between video frame sequences and scale variations in the objects to be recognized, this solution achieves a good balance between speed and accuracy. The validity of the pipeline has been demonstrated on the Trauma THOMPSON dataset, achieving a Mean Average Precision at Intersection over Union threshold of 0.5 (mAP50) of 73.25%. The investigation shows that an adapted, data-driven methodology is more important than the blanket application of general models to specialized areas such as surgical computer vision. The code leading to this solution is available for access via https://github.com/KostasGeorgas97/The-Trauma-THOMPSON-Challenge-2025-Task-2-Hand-Tracking-.

Keywords: Hand Tracking · Surgical Computer Vision · Data-Driven Methodology · YOLOv8 · Object Detection · MICCAI Challenge

1 Introduction

The integration of artificial intelligence into the operating room holds great promise for enhancing surgical efficiency, trainability and patient safety [25]. The core of this paradigm is the interpretation of the surgical scene in real time, with instrument and hand tracking representing fundamental enabling technologies [18]. Automatic recognition of the surgeon's tools and hands enables an

J. P. Wachs et al. (Eds.): TrackRAD/TTC 2025, LNCS 16474, pp. 101–113, 2027.
https://doi.org/10.1007/978-3-032-35046-6_10

intelligent system to provide contextual feedback, automate documentation and control medical tools via gestures [32]. Recent advancements in computer vision and deep learning have facilitated developments in this field, with applications ranging from surgical skill evaluation to autonomous robotic guidance [11]. The Trauma THOMPSON Challenge 2025 [1] focuses specifically on this area with a task for tracking instruments and gloved hands in videos captured during emergency surgical interventions.

Automated tracking is complicated in emergency surgical settings by a number of factors. Classical computer vision systems have significant issues due to the rapid movements associated with trauma therapies, numerous inter-object occlusions, and the visual similarities between gloved hands and instruments [7]. Moreover, the surgical environment carries distinctive domain-specific limitations, such as high sterility standards, restricted computational resources in clinical contexts, and demand for real-time processing capabilities [4,19].

This realization also led to the foundation of this strategic framework: a highly data-driven workflow. In contrast to approaches that rely solely on advances in the architectural improvement of a model, this work instead focuses on a customized pipeline that begins with an exploratory analysis of the problem's dataset. The exploratory data analysis informed all subsequent decisions, including the data curation and preprocessing procedures and the final parameters for model training and inference. The key contributions include:

1. A systematic approach initialized with a comprehensive exploration of the data to enable model building and training by analyzing underlying characteristics, distribution, and potential sources of variability.
2. An optimized and data-informed image processing pipeline with frame skipping to increase training speed and minimize model size.
3. Utilization and configuration of a YOLOv8 model for the accurate and efficient object detection for real-time surgical procedures. The proposed methodology achieved second place in the Trauma THOMPSON Challenge competition.

2 Related Work

2.1 Real-Time Object Detection

Single-stage object detectors have become standard for real-time applications. The YOLO (You Only Look Once) model family ranging from its very first version [29] to later versions including YOLOv8 [16] has consistently challenged the limits of precision and speed. In order to directly predict bounding boxes and class probabilities in a single network pass, these models treat frame detection as a regression problem. Primary architectural components such as the CSPDarknet backbone [39] and the Path Aggregation Network (PANet) neck [22], providing multi-scale feature fusion contribute significantly to their success. Other methods based on deep learning have also been used for object detection. Faster RCNN [30] one of the state-of-the-art methods for object detection, has demonstrated strong performance; however, its two-stage procedure is more computationally expensive than YOLO. In this work, the highly optimized and efficient YOLOv8 architecture is utilized as the baseline framework.

2.2 Computer Vision in Surgery

Computer vision has been applied to a broad range of surgical problems including the observation of surgical workflow analysis [37], instrument segmentation [31,36], and assessment of surgery skills [14]. Databases such as EndoVis [2] and Cholec80 [13] were beneficial in advancing this field of research. Hand tracking is especially critical to understanding the actions of surgeons. Previously, YOLO v10 and v11 based detectors were used in surgical tool detection in instrument images for robotic surgical assistance [6]. Recent work examined the real-time recognition of surgical instruments from operating room footage using Faster R-CNN and Mask R-CNN frameworks, achieving a good trade-off between accuracy and speed [20]. Videos of laparoscopic surgery have commonly been a focus for the detection of AI-driven tools. For example, an improved YOLOv5 algorithm that integrates feature extraction and fusion utilizing mathematical operations and hybrid attention mechanisms was suggested for the real-time identification of surgical instruments [33]. Prior research has investigated the use of both RGB-based tracking techniques [9] as well as depth-based strategies [9]; nevertheless, monitoring gloved hands in a distracting environment continues to be an ongoing challenge [11]. In this regard, a framework combining Faster R-CNN, ResNet-18 and LSTM was employed for classifying hand movements to differentiate visually similar surgical instruments in open surgery [34]. Moreover, a real-time hand tracking system for surgical reasons integrated hand localization, segmentation, and keypoint identification using YOLOv5 and EfficientNet models [26]. In the context of RGB video, the current study offers a practical and highly efficient solution to that particular issue.

2.3 Data-Centric AI Methodologies

In the case of data-centric AI, methodical adjustments to preprocessing and data quality result in more significant advances in a model's performance than model-centric enhancements alone [15]. These include techniques like error analysis, augmentation with resilience, and intelligent data sampling. Frame subsampling, for instance, is a useful technique for video data that strikes a balance between computational expense and semantic integrity [17]. Some additional approaches used in this methodology include letterbox resizing and mosaic augmentation [3], which increase the model's robustness and support for diverse input image dimensions. Data-driven methods for object detection across different image categories, like natural scenes, have demonstrated great potential in tackling issues such as class imbalance, annotation inconsistencies, and limited diversity, thus improving overall data quality and the model's performance [27]. The entire process of the data management and training pipeline is supported by a comprehensive methodology, which includes data analysis throughout.

3 Methods

3.1 Stage 1: Exploratory Data Analysis (EDA)

To understand the Trauma THOMPSON dataset's structural features, content distribution, along with potential biases, the methodological framework starts with a comprehensive exploratory data analysis (EDA), including the following characteristics:

1. Video Properties: Frame rate, resolution, and duration.
2. Annotation Statistics: distribution of left/right hands, number of hands visible in each frame, percentage of frames with annotations.
3. Bounding Box Attributes: Distribution with respect to area of bounding boxes.

Class distribution patterns and bounding box dimensions varied significantly, with several hand instances taking up significant amounts of the native 1920×1080 frame resolution, according to the research. These insights are summarized in Fig. 1.

3.2 Stage 2: Optimized Data Preprocessing Pipeline

To convert the raw video data into a YOLOv8 trainable format, an efficient data preparation pipeline was developed under the direction of the exploratory data analysis (EDA).

1. **VFrame Sub-sampling:** Processing each frame would be computationally demanding and deliver redundant information due to high frame rates and the large number of videos. In order to produce an extensive while manageable set, one frame out of every three was processed, using a frame skipping strategy of two.
2. **Image Padding and Resizing:** As revealed in the exploratory data analysis, hands frequently ended up being large. A target image size of 832×832 pixels was selected in order to maintain clarity at a lower computational cost. To ensure compatibility for the native 16:9 aspect ratio image, a letterboxing scheme was utilized. The image was resized to fit into the 832×832 canvas with an aspect ratio preservation such that the remaining area is filled with a grey value (114, 114, 114) [16]. Geometric distortion of the hands is therefore prevented.
3. **Partitioning of Dataset:** Videos were randomly shuffled and split at the individual video level into a training (80%) and a validation (20%) set. This strategy ensures that frames from a single video do not accidentally appear in both sets and help in a better evaluation of generalization.
4. **Annotation Conversions:** Coordinates of bounding boxes were converted to YOLO format (`class_id, x_center, y_center, width, height`), normalized in proportion to final padded image size.

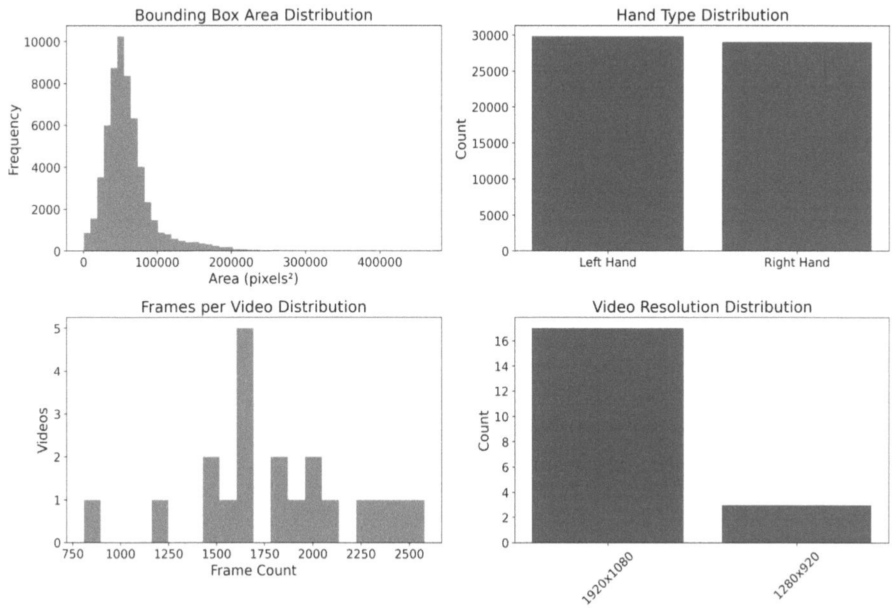

Fig. 1. Exploratory data analysis of the Trauma THOMPSON Challenge 2025 dataset. (a) Bounding box area distribution exhibits right-skewed characteristics, with most hand instances occupying small to moderate spatial extents while a substantial subset encompasses larger frame regions. (b) Hand type distribution demonstrates approximate balance between left and right hand classifications (approximately 27,000 instances each). (c) Frame count distribution across video sequences reveals considerable variability, with most videos containing 1,500–2,000 frames. (d) Video resolution distribution indicates predominant use of 1920 × 1080 pixel footage with a minor subset at lower resolution.

3.3 Stage 3: Model Architecture

The YOLOv8-Large (YOLOv8-L) architecture, that contains over 11.2 million parameters and provides an optimal balance between computational efficiency and detection accuracy, was selected as the detection framework [16]. The four primary components of the architectural pipeline, demonstrated in Fig. 2, perform sequentially.

Input Processing Layer. RGB surgical video frames with a resolution of 832 × 832 × 3 pixels are passed in the input stage. The preprocessing steps and configurations were selected based on the EDA previously presented.

Feature Extraction Backbone. A modified CSPDarknet (Cross Stage Partial Darknet) network using EfficientRep blocks is used in the backbone architecture [38]. By using split methods to divide gradient flow, this design concept improves repetition of features and minimizes computing redundancy. Through

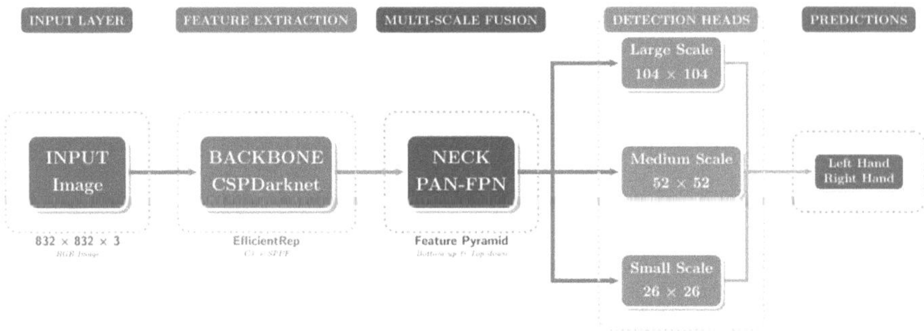

Fig. 2. YOLOv8 architecture for surgical hand detection. The pipeline consists of: (1) Input Layer (832 × 832 × 3 RGB frames), (2) CSPDarknet Backbone with EfficientRep blocks for hierarchical feature extraction, (3) PAN-FPN Neck for multi-scale feature fusion, and (4) Three parallel Detection Heads (104 × 104, 52 × 52, 26 × 26) producing binary hand classifications (left/right) and bounding boxes.

a sequence of convolutional layers grouped into C3 modules, each consisting of many bottleneck blocks with residual connections, the backbone gradually downsamples input features. The architecture results in a Spatial Pyramid Pooling Fast (SPPF) module that allows the network to capture objects at various scales within a computationally efficient framework by aggregating multi-scale contextual information through parallel max-pooling operations with kernel sizes of 5 × 5, 9 × 9, and 13 × 13 [12].

Three feature maps are generated by the hierarchical feature extraction process at progressively lower spatial resolutions (1/8, 1/16, and 1/32 of the input dimensions), each of which retains the capacity to localize spatially while encoding increasingly abstract semantic information.

Multi-Scale Feature Fusion Neck. The neck architecture facilitates bidirectional feature propagation over multiple scales by employing a Path Aggregation Network with Feature Pyramid Network (PAN-FPN) structure [21,22]. Top-down pathway processing is executed by the FPN component, which uses lateral connections and upsampling to transfer semantically powerful characteristics from deeper layers to shallower layers. On the other hand, by propagating spatially accurate features from shallow layers to deep layers, the PAN component performs bottom-up augmentation, enhancing localization information.

Detection Heads and Prediction Output. Three parallel, anchor-free heads employed in resolutions of 104 × 104, 52 × 52, and 26 × 26 for large, medium, and small object dimensions, respectively, comprise the detecting stage. To improve training stability, YOLOv8 adopts a decoupled head architecture with distinct convolutional branches for classification and regression [10]. In order to provide reliable detection throughout the broad variety of hand sizes in surgical procedures, each head outputs precision scores, bounding box coordinates (x, y, w, h), and binary class probabilities (left/right hand) at every spatial position.

Non-Maximum Suppression (NMS) with an IoU threshold of 0.45 is used to aggregate and process the outputs from all three heads [5]. For the purpose of maximizing the precision-recall ratio, a confidence threshold of 0.3 was applied. Final predictions for each detected hand instance includes bounding box coordinates, confidence scores, and class labels.

3.4 Stage 4: Inference

The model utilizes a 0.3 confidence threshold to recognize objects in each input video frame during inference. In order to preserve all true positives while reducing false positives, that threshold was selected. The detected bounding boxes and their class labels of either 'left' or 'right' are then formatted into the required structure.

4 Experiments and Results

4.1 Dataset and Implementation Details

All experiments were conducted on the Trauma THOMPSON Challenge 2025 [41] task 2 training dataset, which consists of 20 videos. Each frame includes manually verified hand-bounding boxes annotated in COCO format. An example image with its corresponding hand bounding boxes is shown in Fig. 3. The initial training set was partitioned into training and validation subsets with an 80/20 split, as described previously.

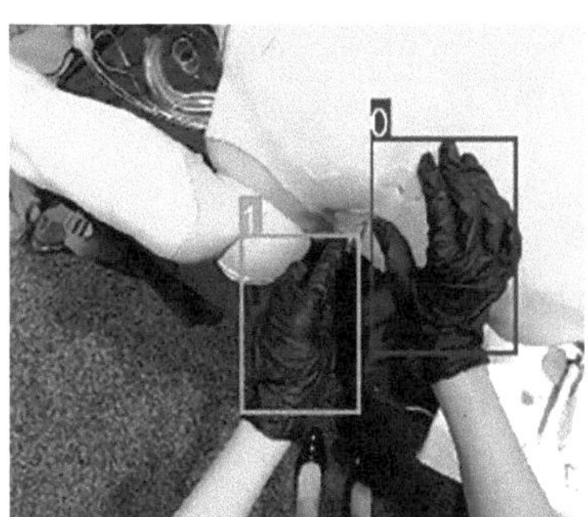

Fig. 3. Dataset example: An image is presented with the ground truth bounding boxes for the hands.

The pipeline was implemented in Python 3 using PyTorch and the Ultralytics framework [16]. Training was performed on an NVIDIA RTX 4090 GPU. A summary of the key training hyperparameters can be found in Table 1.

Table 1. Key training hyperparameters for the YOLOv8-L model in emergency procedure hand tracking.

Parameter	Value	Justification
Model	YOLOv8-L	Largest variant providing superior detection accuracy for critical emergency applications [16]
Image Size	832 × 832	Informed by EDA of large hand objects in emergency procedure contexts
Epochs	100	Sufficient for convergence; model achieved optimal performance at epoch 48
Batch Size	8	Optimized for GPU memory constraints with larger model architecture (RTX 2060 12GB)
Optimizer	AdamW	Standard optimizer with weight decay regularization [24]
Initial LR (lr0)	0.01	Ultralytics recommended default learning rate [16]
Scheduler	Cosine Annealing	Gradual learning rate reduction proven to improve convergence [23]
Mosaic Aug.	1.0 (for 100 epochs)	Multi-image augmentation technique that improves model robustness [3]
Horizontal Flip (fliplr)	0.5	Balances left/right hand classes and improves model generalization [35]
Patience	20	Early stopping threshold if validation loss plateaus for 20 consecutive epochs
Confidence Thresh.	0.3	Empirically determined balance for precision/recall trade-off in hand detection

4.2 Results

To thoroughly evaluate the model's performance and compare it with state-of-the-art object detection models based on YOLO architecture, multiple metrics were employed. Precision quantifies the proportion of true positive detections against all predicted positives while Recall measures the proportion of true positives detected among all actual objects. Mean Average Precision (mAP) is the mean of Average Precision (AP) values across all object classes, with mAP50 referring specifically to the case where the IoU threshold is set to 0.5 and mAP50-95 where averaging AP is performed over multiple IoU thresholds (mAP50-95) [28].

This data-driven methodology produced a highly effective model, securing 2nd place in the challenge. The quantitative performance on the validation set is presented in Table 2. Among models, YOLO8-L achieved the best detection performance with the highest values in three out of four metrics, mAP50 of

0.7325, mAP50-95 of 0.2987 and Recall 0.7041. The high recall value indicates that the model demonstrates strong sensitivity, whereas the high precision value shows that the number of false positives remains low. Although YOLO11-N achieved a precision value higher by 0.5 points compared to YOLO8-L, its low recall value indicates that it failed to detect many objects. The strong performance of YOLO8-S and YOLO8-M supports their suitability for scenarios that require lighter and faster models without a significant loss in accuracy. The results validate our hypothesis that a pipeline tailored to the data's specific characteristics is crucial for achieving top-tier performance.

Table 2. Performance comparison of YOLO variants on emergency procedure hand tracking. Best values are highlighted in bold.

Model	mAP50	mAP50-95	Precision	Recall
YOLOv8-L	**0.7325**	**0.2987**	0.8231	**0.7041**
YOLOv8-S	0.7119	0.2937	0.7846	0.6979
YOLOv8-M	0.7105	0.2911	0.7879	0.6875
YOLOv11-N	0.6979	0.2866	**0.8281**	0.6458
YOLOv11-S	0.6873	0.2866	0.7765	0.6771
YOLOv8-N	0.6743	0.2801	0.8090	0.6250
YOLOv11-L	0.6231	0.2414	0.7302	0.5938
YOLOv11-M	0.5084	0.1940	0.5843	0.5104

Figure 4 illustrates a baseline example where the ground truth labels are compared with the predictions of the proposed methodology. In all four frames, the proposed model correctly identified both hands. Moreover, in three of the four frames, the predicted bounding boxes closely matched the ground truth, while in the last frame, the model underestimated the bounding box, producing a smaller one.

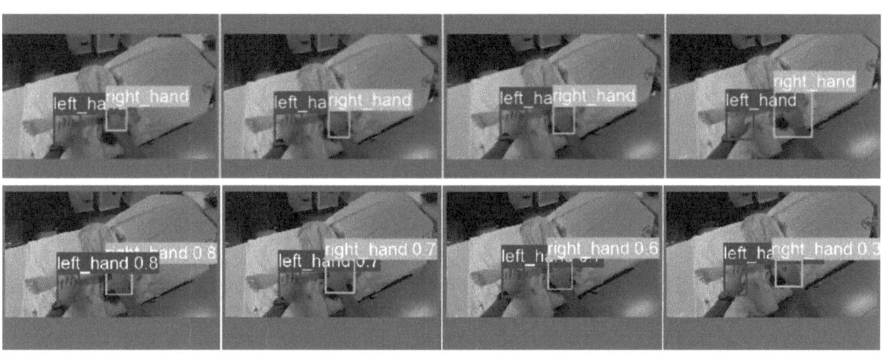

Fig. 4. Qualitative example showing successful hand tracking. **Top row:** Ground truth annotations **Bottom row:** Model predictions with confidence scores.

5 Discussion

Remote systems based on artificial intelligence can provide real-time guidance during medical procedures in resource-limited settings. A crucial first step in these systems is the reliable identification of the environment and relevant objects from videos streams. Detecting objects, such as hands and tools remains challenging due to variations objects' appearance, scenes' complexity and real-time requirements. Accurate hand tracking is important for identifying and guiding the users' actions. In this work, a pipeline based on data analysis and object detection techniques is proposed to enable robust hand detection from egocentric video captured in emergency medical procedures.

The decision to utilize an extended input resolution of 832 × 832 pixels, directly informed by our exploratory data analysis (EDA), proved critical to the model's performance. By mitigating the aggressive downsampling common in standard configurations, this resolution preserved essential semantic details and improved the detection of hand instances across varying spatial scales, particularly in cases of occlusion or smaller relative object size. Utilizing every video frame during training typically introduces redundancy and increases computational demands. Our frame-skipping strategy was crucial to successful training over the large-sized video dataset by allowing us to preserve a wide variety of training instances.

As it is presented in related works, many architectures, e.g. Mask RCNN, Faster R-CNN, have been previously proposed for object detection in video sequences. Our work integrates YOLOv8, a state-of-the-art object detection model, into a customized pipeline to implement a data-oriented AI methodology for better training and thus higher accuracy. YOLOv8 was selected for its excellent trade-off between accuracy and speed which is crucial in real-time detection frameworks. It employs a one-stage procedure that produces dense predictions directly, in contrast to two-stage pipelines that perform region localization and classification separately. Though the YOLOv8 model has immense potential, putting it to common use could not have produced similar outcomes without the specially customized data processing pipeline that we assembled. The training procedure of YOLOv8 is sensitive to redundant frames, class imbalance, and domain-specific properties, which can otherwise lead to biased predictions and poor generalization. The data-driven framework proposed in this work is designed and implemented to address these challenges and enhance training.

There are, however, certain limitations in the proposed work that can be addressed in future research. While a limitation of this study is the lack of explicit temporal modeling, YOLO-based detection techniques operate on separate frames, prioritizing real-time inference speed over temporal consistency. Future research endeavors can implement tracking algorithms such as DeepSORT [40] or incorporate a temporal model such as a Vision Transformer [8] to boost frame-to-frame consistency and, at times of intense, brief occlusion, potentially augmenting robustness. Secondly, the aspect of tool recognition in our task was omitted from our decisive model, yet it is possible that it can be included as another classification head.

6 Conclusion

In this paper, an overview of the data-driven methodology that facilitated the second-place ranking in the Trauma THOMPSON Challenge 2025 for hand tracking is presented. In order to create a customized preprocessing and training pipeline that optimized a YOLOv8-L model for the particular challenges of the surgical video dataset, the study started with a comprehensive analysis of the data. The experiments that were conducted confirm this process as an effective approach, demonstrating that a thorough understanding of the data is essential for tuning the training. Although no fundamental architectural changes were made to the YOLOv8 backbone, the significant performance gains achieved solely through this data-centric application strategy highlight that domain-specific preprocessing is often more critical than architectural novelty in surgical computer vision.

Author contributions. The authors declare contributions in accordance with the CRediT (Contributor Roles Taxonomy):
- **Konstantinos Georgas (PhD Candidate)**: Conceptualization; Methodology; Software; Validation; Formal Analysis; Investigation; Resources; Data Curation; Writing Original Draft; Writing Review & Editing; Visualization; Writing Review & Editing.
- **Theodoros P. Vagenas (PhD Candidate)**: Conceptualization; Methodology; Software; Validation; Formal Analysis; Investigation; Resources; Data Curation; Writing Original Draft; Writing Review & Editing; Visualization; Writing Review & Editing.
- **Prof. George K. Matsopoulos**: Supervision; Project Administration.

Other Information. The authors state that there was no external funding or institutional collaboration that contributed to this work. There are no competing interests.

References

1. Trauma thompson challenge 2025: Tracking hands and objects in major polytrauma surgery (2025). https://t3challenge25.grand-challenge.org/
2. Allan, M., et al.: 2018 robotic scene segmentation challenge. arXiv preprint arXiv:2001.11190 (2020)
3. Bochkovskiy, A., Wang, C.Y., Liao, H.Y.M.: Yolov4: optimal speed and accuracy of object detection. arXiv preprintarXiv:2004.10934 (2020)
4. Bodenstedt, S., et al.: Prediction of laparoscopic procedure duration using unlabeled, multimodal sensor data. Int. J. Comput. Assist. Radiol. Surg. **14**(6), 1089–1095 (2019)
5. Bodla, N., Singh, B., Chellappa, R., Davis, L.S.: Soft-NMS-improving object detection with one line of code. In: Proceedings of the IEEE International Conference on Computer Vision, pp. 5561–5569 (2017)
6. Chellamani, G.K., N, A., P, B.K., Reddy, P.S.K., Babu, R.T.S.: A robust dataset for surgical instrument detection to aid autonomous robotic surgery. Data Brief **61**, 111798 (2025). https://doi.org/10.1016/J.DIB.2025.111798

7. Daneshgar Rahbar, M., Pappas, G., Jaber, N.: Toward intraoperative visual intelligence: real-time surgical instrument segmentation for enhanced surgical monitoring. In: Healthcare, vol. 12, p. 1112. MDPI (2024)
8. Dosovitskiy, A., et al.: An image is worth 16x16 words: transformers for image recognition at scale. arXiv preprint arXiv:2010.11929 (2020)
9. Ge, L., et al.: 3d hand shape and pose estimation from a single RGB image. In: Proceedings of the IEEE/CVF Conference on Computer Vision and Pattern Recognition, pp. 10833–10842 (2019)
10. Ge, Z., Liu, S., Wang, F., Li, Z., Sun, J.: Yolox: exceeding yolo series in 2021. arXiv preprint arXiv:2107.08430 (2021)
11. Guni, A., Varma, P., Zhang, J., Fehervari, M., Ashrafian, H.: Artificial intelligence in surgery: the future is now. Eur. Surg. Res. **65**(1), 22–39 (2024)
12. He, K., Zhang, X., Ren, S., Sun, J.: Spatial pyramid pooling in deep convolutional networks for visual recognition. IEEE Trans. Pattern Anal. Mach. Intell. **37**(9), 1904–1916 (2015)
13. Hong, W.Y., Kao, C.L., Kuo, Y.H., Wang, J.R., Chang, W.L., Shih, C.S.: Cholecseg8k: a semantic segmentation dataset for laparoscopic cholecystectomy based on cholec80. arXiv preprint arXiv:2012.12453 (2020)
14. Igaki, T., et al.: Automatic surgical skill assessment system based on concordance of standardized surgical field development using artificial intelligence. JAMA Surg. **158**(8), e231131–e231131 (2023)
15. Jakubik, J., Vössing, M., Kühl, N., Walk, J., Satzger, G.: Data-centric artificial intelligence. Bus. Inf. Syst. Eng. **66**(4), 507–515 (2024)
16. Jocher, G., Chaurasia, A., Qiu, J.: Yolo by ultralytics (2023)
17. Karpathy, A., Toderici, G., Shetty, S., Leung, T., Sukthankar, R., Fei-Fei, L.: Large-scale video classification with convolutional neural networks. In: Proceedings of the IEEE Conference on Computer Vision and Pattern Recognition, pp. 1725–1732 (2014)
18. Kenngott, H., et al.: Computer-assisted abdominal surgery: new technologies. Langenbecks Arch. Surg. **400**(3), 273–281 (2015)
19. Laina, I., et al.: Concurrent segmentation and localization for tracking of surgical instruments. In: International Conference on Medical Image Computing and Computer-Assisted Intervention, pp. 664–672. Springer, Cham (2017)
20. Lee, J.D., Chien, J.C., Hsu, Y.T., Wu, C.T.: Automatic surgical instrument recognition—a case of comparison study between the faster r-cnn, mask r-cnn, and single-shot multi-box detectors. Appl. Sci. **11**(17) (2021). https://doi.org/10.3390/app11178097, https://www.mdpi.com/2076-3417/11/17/8097
21. Lin, T.Y., Dollár, P., Girshick, R., He, K., Hariharan, B., Belongie, S.: Feature pyramid networks for object detection. In: Proceedings of the IEEE Conference on Computer Vision and Pattern Recognition, pp. 2117–2125 (2017)
22. Liu, S., Qi, L., Qin, H., Shi, J., Jia, J.: Path aggregation network for instance segmentation. In: Proceedings of the IEEE Conference on Computer Vision and Pattern Recognition, pp. 8759–8768 (2018)
23. Loshchilov, I., Hutter, F.: Sgdr: Stochastic gradient descent with warm restarts. arXiv preprint arXiv:1608.03983 (2016)
24. Loshchilov, I., Hutter, F.: Decoupled weight decay regularization. arXiv preprint arXiv:1711.05101 (2017)
25. Maier-Hein, L., et al.: Surgical data science-from concepts toward clinical translation. Med. Image Anal. **76**, 102306 (2022)

26. Müller, L.R., et al.: Robust hand tracking for surgical telestration. Int. J. Comput. Assist. Radiol. Surg. **17**, 1477–1486 (2022). https://doi.org/10.1007/S11548-022-02637-9/FIGURES/7
27. Nayak, R., Pati, U.C., Das, S.K.: A comprehensive review of datasets for detection and localization of video anomalies: a step towards data-centric artificial intelligence-based video anomaly detection. Multimedia Tools Appl. **83**, 59617–59674 (2024). https://doi.org/10.1007/S11042-023-17889-Z/FIGURES/1
28. Padilla, R., Netto, S.L., Da Silva, E.A.: A survey on performance metrics for object-detection algorithms. In: 2020 International Conference on Systems, Signals and Image Processing (IWSSIP), pp. 237–242. IEEE (2020)
29. Redmon, J., Divvala, S., Girshick, R., Farhadi, A.: You only look once: unified, real-time object detection. In: Proceedings of the IEEE Conference on Computer Vision and Pattern Recognition, pp. 779–788 (2016)
30. Ren, S., He, K., Girshick, R., Sun, J.: Faster r-cnn: towards real-time object detection with region proposal networks. In: Advances in Neural Information Processing Systems, vol. 28 (2015). https://github.com/
31. Ross, T., et al.: Robust medical instrument segmentation challenge 2019. arXiv preprint arXiv:2003.10299 (2020)
32. Salvador, R.A., Naval, P.: Towards a feasible hand gesture recognition system as sterile non-contact interface in the operating room with 3d convolutional neural network. Informatica **46**(1) (2022)
33. Shao, Y., Xu, Z., Zhu, Q.: Sh-yolo: enhanced real-time detection of laparoscopic surgical instruments in computer-aided surgery based on star operation and hybrid attention mechanisms. IEEE Access **13**, 135179–135195 (2025). https://doi.org/10.1109/ACCESS.2025.3593635
34. Shimizu, T., Hachiuma, R., Kajita, H., Takatsume, Y., Saito, H.: Hand motion-aware surgical tool localization and classification from an egocentric camera. J. Imaging **7**(2) (2021). https://doi.org/10.3390/jimaging7020015, https://www.mdpi.com/2313-433X/7/2/15
35. Shorten, C., Khoshgoftaar, T.M.: A survey on image data augmentation for deep learning. J. Big Data **6**(1), 1–48 (2019)
36. Shvets, A.A., Rakhlin, A., Kalinin, A.A., Iglovikov, V.I.: Automatic instrument segmentation in robot-assisted surgery using deep learning. In: 17th IEEE International Conference on Machine Learning and Applications (ICMLA), pp. 624–628. IEEE (2018)
37. Twinanda, A.P., Shehata, S., Mutter, D., Marescaux, J., De Mathelin, M., Padoy, N.: Endonet: a deep architecture for recognition tasks on laparoscopic videos. IEEE Trans. Med. Imaging **36**(1), 86–97 (2016)
38. Wang, C.Y., Bochkovskiy, A., Liao, H.Y.M.: Yolov7: trainable bag-of-freebies sets new state-of-the-art for real-time object detectors. In: Proceedings of the IEEE/CVF Conference on Computer Vision and Pattern Recognition, pp. 7464–7475 (2023)
39. Wang, C.Y., Liao, H.Y.M., Wu, Y.H., Chen, P.Y., Hsieh, J.W., Yeh, I.H.: Cspnet: a new backbone that can enhance learning capability of CNN. In: Proceedings of the IEEE/CVF Conference on Computer Vision and Pattern Recognition Workshops, pp. 390–391 (2020)
40. Wojke, N., Bewley, A., Paulus, D.: Simple online and realtime tracking with a deep association metric. In: 2017 IEEE International Conference on Image Processing (ICIP), pp. 3645–3649. IEEE (2017)
41. Zhuo, Y., et al.: An egocentric life-saving interventional procedure dataset of actions, medical questions, maneuvers and tools. Sci. Data (2025)

A Lifesaving Foundation: Leveraging Foundation Models for Recognizing and Anticipating Medical Procedure Actions

Adrian Leon Lindloff[1(✉)], Simone Frintrop[1], Christian Wilms[1(✉)], and Matthias Wilms[2]

[1] Computer Vision Group, University of Hamburg, Hamburg, Germany
al.lindloff01@gmail.com, {simone.frintrop,christian.wilms}@uni-hamburg.de
[2] Department of Radiology, University of Michigan, Ann Arbor, USA
wilms@umich.edu

Abstract. First responders play a pivotal role in medical emergency situations, where timely and accurate decision-making can be lifesaving. To provide support in such scenarios, computer vision-based systems with the ability to recognize the currently ongoing procedure and anticipate the next steps are of significant interest, as they could assist in guiding first responders through critical interventions. However, annotated data to train such systems is scarce. Therefore, we study the applicability of recent foundation models on the tasks of recognizing and anticipating medical procedure actions from video data as part of The Trauma THOMPSON Challenge 2025. Specifically, we adapt image-based DINOv2, video-based VideoMAE, and multi-modal ActionCLIP to the problem by adjusting prompt handling, hyperparameters, and loss weighting. In our evaluation, we show that despite the limited amount of training data in the challenge dataset, the models are able to achieve moderate performance in recognizing medical procedure actions, particularly under simpler evaluation criteria on the validation data.

Keywords: Action Recognition · Action Anticipation · Life-Saving Interventions (LSI) · Foundation Models · Video Classification

1 Introduction

In medical emergencies, first responders play a critical role and often dictate the outcome regarding not just the immediate, but also the long-term future of a patient [11]. First responders need to quickly identify the precise characteristics of such situations and perform the appropriate medical treatment under immense pressure. Support from an experienced assistant can substantially improve the

C. Wilms and M. Wilms—Shared senior authorship.

J. P. Wachs et al. (Eds.): TrackRAD/TTC 2025, LNCS 16474, pp. 114–125, 2027.
https://doi.org/10.1007/978-3-032-35046-6_11

quality; however, such support is rarely available due to the nature of these situations. Therefore, computer vision-based autonomous remote instruction systems are envisioned to mitigate the lack of human assistance.

With this goal in mind, the Trauma THOMPSON Challenge 2025 [23,24] was proposed to facilitate the development of such systems for lifesaving interventions. The challenge introduces a first-person video dataset of unscripted emergency interventions to foster the development of algorithms that can recognize and anticipate medical procedures, detect tools, and track hand movements during an intervention, assess the realism of a simulated trauma procedure, and perform visual clinical question answering. Here, we focus on the recognition and prediction of medical procedure actions, both tasks that are closely related to general action recognition in computer vision. While action recognition refers to assigning an action to the currently analyzed video part, action prediction involves forecasting the action of the subsequent video part.

Over the years, many approaches have been proposed to address the video action recognition task. First, before public video datasets of sufficient size existed, methods such as cuboids [7] relied on traditional feature engineering to design hand-crafted spatio-temporal representations to detect actions. Using deep learning, architectures evolved to be more automated and, among other techniques, (1) extract per frame features through 2D CNNs [19], also with an additional LSTM on top [8], (2) apply 3D CNNs directly to videos [4,18], (3) extract spatial and temporal features individually with two-stream networks [10], or more recently, (4) apply vision transformers (ViTs) [9] to the video classification problem [1]. In recent years, foundation models have substantially improved the performance across various computer vision domains, including video-related tasks such as video classification [2,21]. Due to their extensive training on huge amounts of data, foundation models are able to generate rich general-purpose features, allowing them to generalize well to a wide range of tasks without extensive training data. This makes foundation models highly suitable for tasks where data is expensive or difficult to acquire, like in medical applications [14].

In this paper, we adapt three well-known foundation models: DINOv2 [15], VideoMAE [17], and ActionCLIP [20], to the task of medical procedure action recognition and anticipation in the context of the Trauma THOMPSON (T3) Challenge 2025. Foundation models with their strong few-shot capabilities [2] may be particularly well-suited for the setting of the 2025 T3 Challenge, which features 124 classes in a long-tailed distribution across 2477 training samples. The three selected foundation models cover a variety of input modalities, including images, video, and text (see Fig. 2), which allows us to study the effect of these modalities. To adapt the foundation models for the dual-task formulation, we incorporate video action classifiers for the recognition and anticipation tasks when necessary. In our evaluation of the 2025 T3 Challenge data, the three models with tailored prompt handling, hyperparameters, and loss weighting demonstrate promising results.

2 Dataset

The T3 Challenge 2025 dataset [24], which we use in this work, is an egocentric video dataset specifically built for medical procedure action recognition and anticipation. For this task, corresponding to task 1 in the challenge, it comprises 141 videos of regular life-saving intervention procedures in its training set and another 79 videos in the test set. The test set is further split into 36 unseen regular procedure videos and 43 just-in-time procedure videos. Each video presents a medical procedure and consists of several shorter video clips, representing individual actions. In total, the training dataset consists of 2477 video clips. On average, a single video clip consists of around 152 frames, and the original resolution of the video clips is 1920×1080. Following the official challenge instructions, we resized the video clips to 480×270 pixels.

Each video clip is annotated with an action label that represents the action currently performed. A label consists of one verb and one noun, each of which can individually reappear in other action labels. Each clip annotation also contains the action label of the subsequent video clip. In total, there are 124 action classes in the training set, composed of 42 unique nouns and 42 distinct verb classes. The class distribution represents the real-world distribution of the procedures, similar to how the procedures themselves were chosen to reflect relevant medical interventions. This leads to a long-tailed class distribution, as illustrated in Fig. 1. As a consequence, a few common action classes dominate a significant number of minority classes. For reference, the most frequent action 'insert finger' appears in 85 video clips, while a multitude of actions only appear a single time.

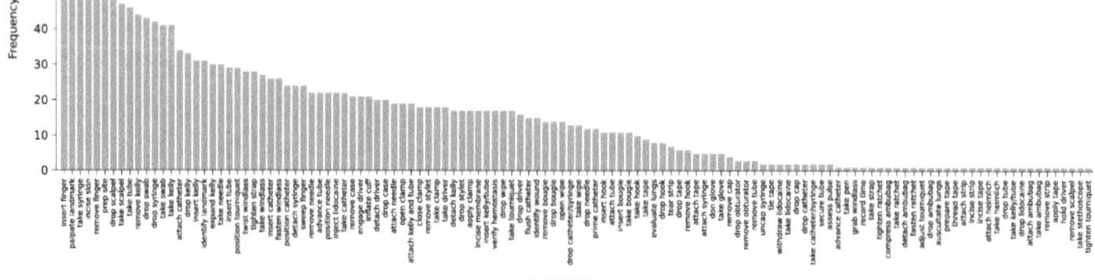

Fig. 1. Distribution of action classes (combinations of nouns and verbs) in the training set of the T3 Challenge 2025 dataset, with actions on the x-axis and frequency on the y-axis.

For our work, we split the original training set into our training set (80%) and our validation set (20%). Hence, 1968 video clips remain for the training. Due to the considerable class imbalance, 16 of the 124 action classes occur only once and can not occur in both sets. To enable the model to learn from all classes, these samples are added to our training set. Consequently, our validation set only includes 108 action classes.

3 Method

This section introduces our adapted versions of the three foundation models, which we employ for action recognition and anticipation (task 1) of the T3 Challenge 2025. For each model, we discuss the architecture, as shown in Fig. 2, and the implementation details[1]. The presented model configurations are based on the best-performing results obtained through extensive evaluation on the 2023 T3 Challenge dataset.

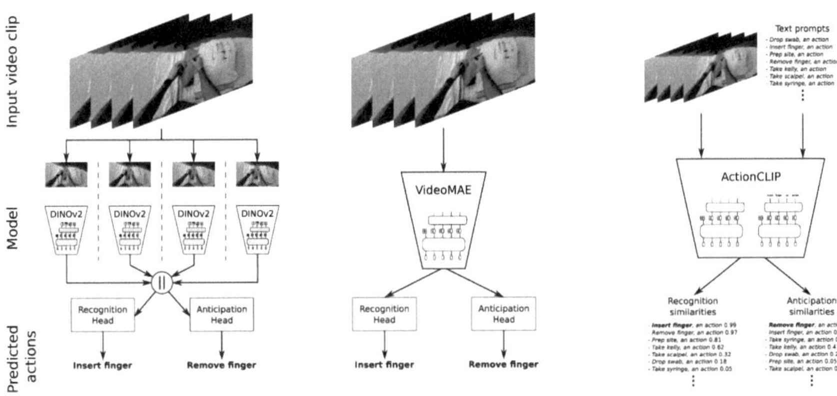

(a) DINOv2 (b) VideoMAE (c) ActionCLIP

Fig. 2. General processing of videos for action recognition and anticipation with the three foundation models. Image-based DINOv2 (a) processes individual frames and combines the results in the final stage. Video-based VideoMAE (b) directly extracts features from the entire video clip with subsequent classification. Multi-modal Action-CLIP (c) extracts features from the entire video and the label via text prompt. Subsequently, classification is performed as a similarity calculation between a video and all possible text prompt representations.

3.1 DINOv2

DINOv2 [15] is a discriminative self-supervised learning approach, which produces general-purpose visual features for images. Besides other computer vision tasks, DINOv2 was successfully applied to video action recognition tasks outside the medical domain [15]. Among self-supervised approaches at the time

[1] https://github.com/Loffl/A-Lifesaving-Foundation-The-Trauma-THOMPSON-Challenge-2025-solution.

of its publication, DINOv2 achieved state-of-the-art accuracy performance even though the model was trained on images only. Therefore, we adapt DINOv2 to the T3 Challenge 2025.

Architecture. The DINOv2 [15] learning approach combines the ideas of DINO [3] and iBOT [22]. DINO [3] works at the image-level, after obtaining features from the ViT backbone. It utilizes a student-teacher architecture, where each receives a different crop of the same image as input to generate a ViT class token. Each token is forwarded to the respective head for loss calculation.

The iBOT method [22] is employed at the patch-level and thus alters the input behavior of the ViT model. The input image patches are randomly masked and distributed to the same student and teacher model. The student operates on the masked patches, whereas the teacher employs the entire tokenized image without any masks, enabling the teacher to process information unavailable to the student network. The output features are passed to the corresponding student and teacher iBOT MLP head to produce the loss.

At first, both the DINO and iBOT methods are strictly separated from each other as they compute their own losses. Their knowledge is only brought together when both losses of a given batch are combined with a regularization term to train the student model. After the pre-training has been completed, only the student network is used to generate image representations.

To apply DINOv2 to video action recognition, we obtain the output embeddings for each frame as depicted in Fig. 2a. The classification (`CLS`) tokens, as well as the remaining embedding sequences of all frame representations for a sample, are averaged and then concatenated to imitate video representations. These are forwarded to two linear classification heads for recognition and anticipation, respectively, as illustrated in the lower section of Fig. 2a. The Cross-Entropy Loss is applied to the resulting logits to compute the action losses.

Concerning anticipation, only valid samples are considered for the loss computation. A sample is not valid when there is no next action present, in case it is the last clip of a video. Both the recognition and the anticipation losses are combined to form a final action loss, which, in the simplest case, is obtained by weighting them equally. In our experiments, we investigate the impact of different loss weighting methods on the model's performance.

Implementation Details. For the application of DINOv2, we first uniformly sample 16 frames for each video clip. Next, each frame is randomly cropped and resized to 224×224. A higher resolution is not possible when using the pre-trained model weights. The frames are horizontally flipped with a 50% probability and randomly rotated by up to two degrees, before being scaled by a factor between 0.8 and 1.2. The validation and test data are only uniformly sampled and resized.

The following parameters were utilized for our DINOv2 experiments on the 2025 T3 Challenge dataset. The batch size is set to 20, and training lasts for 50 epochs. Gradient clipping is enabled and set to 1.0. For the optimizer, AdamW is employed with a β_1 of 0.9, a β_2 of 0.999, and $\epsilon = 10^{-8}$. Weight decay is set to 0.1, and the learning rate is initialized at 5×10^{-5}. It is controlled by a cosine annealing scheduler with a linear warm-up phase over the first 10% of training steps. Gradient accumulation is enabled and fixed at 2, meaning that gradients are accumulated for two forward passes before the weights are updated. We use a large-sized ViT backbone with four additional register tokens. The register tokens [6] have proven to sufficiently remove existing artifacts in the Vision Transformer attention maps.

3.2 VideoMAE

VideoMAE [17] by Tong et al. is a transformer-based foundation model, explicitly designed to process video data (see Fig. 2b) as it extends the concept of masked autoencoders for self-supervised pre-training to videos. Similar to the DINOv2 approach for images, VideoMAE extracts semantically rich general-purpose video representations. Since it is designed to extract features from videos, action recognition constitutes an intuitive application, which Tong et al. briefly explore, reporting state-of-the-art accuracies on relevant benchmarks.

Architecture. Inspired by ImageMAE [12], VideoMAE performs a masking and reconstruction task using an asymmetric encoder-decoder architecture in a self-supervised setup. The encoder is a ViT with joint space-time attention. Before a video is processed by the encoder, uniform temporal downsampling is applied. Subsequently, the video is embedded into 3D tokens using joint space-time cube embedding, which are then mapped to the transformer embedding dimension. Each cube has the size $2 \times 16 \times 16$, meaning it contains spatial patches of two frames. Next, tube masking is applied. Due to the high redundancy in video data, the masking ratio is set between 90% and 95%. The non-masked tokens are used as the input for the encoder.

Given the output representations of the visible tokens from the encoder and the remaining learnable masked tokens, a lightweight ViT-based decoder reconstructs the missing tokens and thus recreates the entire video. This enables VideoMAE to learn meaningful video representations. The generated video representations are processed by two linear classifiers as visualized in the bottom part of Fig. 2b, one for obtaining recognition logits and another for anticipation probabilities when a sample is valid.

Implementation Details. To adapt VideoMAE to the T3 Challenge 2025, we uniformly downsample each video to 16 input frames. We then randomly downsize each frame while maintaining the original aspect ratio and randomly extract crops of size 224×224. Finally, random left-right flipping is applied. Remaining transformations correspond to the DINOv2 data preprocessing. For the validation and test data, only the initial temporal downsampling is applied. Hence, we do not apply test-time augmentation.

The VideoMAE configurations of our experiments adopt the following training parameters. We set the batch size to 2 and train for 50 epochs. There is no weight decay, and the learning rate is set to 5×10^{-5}. The ViT backbone is huge-sized, and no register tokens are utilized. All remaining configuration settings mirror the training method of DINOv2, including the Cross-Entropy Loss.

3.3 ActionCLIP

The CLIP-based [16] model ActionCLIP [20] is a foundation model proposed by Mengmeng Wang et al. It was specifically designed for video action recognition and could thus translate particularly well to the target data. It has outperformed other ViT-based model architectures on the Kinetics-400 [13] action recognition benchmark, setting new state-of-the-art accuracy scores.

Architecture. In contrast to DINOv2 and VideoMAE, which exclusively rely on visual input, ActionCLIP [20] utilizes both visual and text supervision in a multi-modal framework tailored for action recognition. It frames action recognition as a video-text similarity matching problem. To achieve this, ActionCLIP creates distinct representations for the visual and text input using two encoders as depicted in Fig. 2c.

The text encoder is a 12-layer Transformer based on the CLIP architecture [16]. As input prompts for the text encoder, we utilize 16 possible templates for each of the 124 action classes in the 2025 T3 Challenge. Given a label, a prompt is created by replacing a blank field within a template, for example, "`Label`, an action" for the recognition task. When anticipating actions, we apply slightly modified templates such as "`Label`, an upcoming action". During the training, a single text prompt is randomly selected from the 16 available candidates for each video clip and for action recognition and anticipation labels, respectively, which is then fed to the text encoder. For inference, all 16×124 prompts are used for both subtasks, with the most similar prompt indicating the predicted action label, as shown in the bottom part of Fig. 2c, which visualizes this process with seven representative prompts.

The vision encoder in ActionCLIP is a standard ViT-Base with a patch size of 16×16. We use ActionCLIP's post-network prompt to capture temporal relations between different frames. This is accomplished by adding a second, separate vision encoder, which receives the concatenated frame-level representations of the initial pre-trained CLIP vision encoder. The second encoder is a temporal transformer with extra learnable temporal positional embeddings and a mean-pooled output sequence, yielding a feature representation of the entire video.

Given the text and vision representations, ActionCLIP calculates the similarities between them. The idea is to align matching representations, a text prompt that describes the action of the respective video, by pulling the pairwise text and video representations close to each other. This is achieved by computing symmetric cosine similarity scores across all conceivable modality pairs of feature embeddings. The video-to-text similarity scores quantify how similar a given video embedding is to all other text embeddings in the batch, while text-to-video scores capture the reverse relationship.

Implementation Details. To handle the T3 Challenge 2025 video data with ActionCLIP, we split every video clip into 16 segments, from which two consecutive frames are sampled each. We largely follow Wang et al. [20] to pre-process the extracted frames. First, two random image augmentations are applied to each frame, given a pool of 14 possible operations, including geometric, color, and intensity transformations [5]. Subsequently, the frames are cropped randomly at different scales and resized to 224 × 224 pixels. Finally, the frames are horizontally flipped with a probability of 50%, a random color jitter is applied, and 20% of the frames are randomly converted to grayscale. All frames of a video are stacked and provided as input to ActionCLIP. During validation and testing, the frames are only resized and center-cropped. Hence, we do not apply test-time augmentation.

To train ActionCLIP, the Kullback-Leibler (KL) divergence is utilized as a loss function. Given a label y and a paired video clip x, it is calculated once for the video-to-text similarity scores $p^{x2y}(\boldsymbol{x})$ and once for the text-to-video similarity scores $p^{y2x}(\boldsymbol{y})$ of a batch, to create a symmetric contrastive learning objective defined as:

$$\mathcal{L} = \frac{1}{2}\mathbb{E}_{(x,y)\sim\mathcal{T}}\left[\mathrm{KL}\left(\boldsymbol{p}^{x2y}(\boldsymbol{x}), \boldsymbol{q}^{x2y}(\boldsymbol{x})\right) + \mathrm{KL}\left(\boldsymbol{p}^{y2x}(\boldsymbol{y}), \boldsymbol{q}^{y2x}(\boldsymbol{y})\right)\right] \tag{1}$$

where $\mathcal{T}$ denotes the entire training set and $q^{x\ 2y}(x), q^{y2x}(y)$ correspond to the ground-truth similarity scores [20]. Since the recognition and the anticipation tasks employ different text embeddings, we calculate four similarity scores and two losses. We evaluate several strategies to combine the recognition and anticipation losses in Sect. 4.2.

Our ActionCLIP experiments utilize a batch size of 12, the training lasts for 75 epochs, and gradients are clipped when exceeding a value of 20. AdamW is the optimizer, with a β_1 of 0.9, a β_2 of 0.98, and $\epsilon = 10^{-8}$. The weight decay rate is set to 0.2 and the base learning rate to 5×10^{-6}. The post-network prompt is trained with a learning rate set to ten times the base rate. A standard cosine annealing scheduler with a five-step linear warm-up is employed.

4 Results

In this section, we evaluate the three foundation models on the T3 Challenge 2025 dataset to assess their suitability for the action recognition and anticipation tasks. All models and variations are trained on our training set as outlined in Sect. 2 and evaluated on our validation set or the official test set. Top-1 and top-5 accuracies serve as the evaluation metrics for both tasks individually. We also report the average accuracy across both tasks to evaluate the overall performance. Note that on the official test set, only top-1 accuracies are available.

4.1 Loss Weighting

Since task 1 of the 2025 T3 Challenge is formulated as a dual-task problem, consisting of action recognition and anticipation, we compare three strategies for weighting the individual task losses, yielding the overall loss. First, we combine the two losses for action recognition and anticipation by scaling them with 0.5 before adding them. We coin this strategy `Equal`. Second, we progressively adapt the loss weights throughout the training process. Specifically, we start with a higher weight on the recognition loss (0.6) compared to the anticipation loss (0.4) and linearly adjust the weights between epochs such that in the final epoch, we again reach 0.5 for both losses. This strategy is called `Linear` and follows the premise that recognition might be easier to learn initially and, therefore, stronger supervision could result in better shared representations. As our third strategy, we follow Wang et al. [20] and apply the `Equal` strategy, but introduce an additional loss term scaled by a factor that linearly decreases from 0.15 to 0.05 throughout training. The additional loss is a symmetric bidirectional KL Divergence loss, which encourages the model to predict similar distributions for recognition and anticipation, as both actions are often closely related in their temporal context. Hence, we name the strategy `KLD`.

4.2 Results on the Validation Set

Table 1 presents the results of the three foundation models on our validation set. The results of the systems are substantially different between the two tasks. While VideoMAE and DINOv2 consistently outperform ActionCLIP on the action recognition task with top-1 accuracies of 47.74% and 43.22% compared to 40.48%, ActionCLIP excels in action anticipation, achieving a top-1 accuracy of 35.15%. On this task, VideoMAE and DINOv2 only yield 20.04% and 29.67% at best.

Table 1. Results of the three foundation models on our validation set for the T3 Challenge 2025, employing each of our three loss weighting strategies. Top-1 and top-5 accuracies are reported separately for recognition, anticipation, and the combination. Bold font highlights the best overall results, whereas slanted font indicates the best results for each foundation model.

	Loss	Recognition		Anticipation		Total	
Model	Weighting	Top-1	Top-5	Top-1	Top-5	Top-1	Top-5
DINOv2	Equal	42.83%	80.55%	25.34%	76.23%	34.09%	78.39%
VideoMAE	Equal	46.17%	74.66%	13.95%	64.24%	30.06%	69.45%
ActionCLIP	Equal	*40.48%*	*82.74%*	***35.15%***	*82.01%*	***37.82%***	*82.38%*
DINOv2	Linear	41.65%	79.37%	25.15%	76.62%	33.40%	77.99%
VideoMAE	Linear	47.54%	75.83%	13.36%	58.35%	30.45%	67.09%
ActionCLIP	Linear	35.71%	81.94%	33.05%	80.33%	34.38%	81.14%
DINOv2	KLD	*43.22%*	***88.80%***	*29.67%*	***88.61%***	*36.45%*	***88.71%***
VideoMAE	KLD	***47.74%***	*78.19%*	*20.04%*	*76.42%*	*33.89%*	*77.31%*
ActionCLIP	KLD	33.93%	79.96%	33.68%	80.33%	33.81%	80.15%

As expected, these results also indicate that recognizing the current action is generally a simpler task compared to anticipating the next action. Extending the output scope from one prediction to five predictions (top-5 accuracy), DINOv2 produces the best results across both tasks with 88.80% and 88,61%. This is at least 6.1% better than the other two models. Investigating the effect of the three proposed loss weighting strategies shows that VideoMAE and DINOv2 profit from the additional KL Divergence loss of `KLD`, while ActionCLIP performs best when trained with the default equal weighting. The linearly adjusted loss amounts to no measurable improvements.

4.3 Results on the Test Set

We report the results of DINOv2, VideoMAE, and ActionCLIP on the official test set of the T3 Challenge 2025 in Table 2. We selected these model configurations due to the strong performance on the challenge's open development test set. In contrast to the validation data, the official test set includes additional so-called just-in-time procedures intended to increase task difficulty. These procedures were recorded using improvised, unconventional medical tools, such as a belt and a screwdriver in place of a tourniquet. The results in Table 2 indicate that all three models have difficulties generalizing to the new data, especially for the action recognition task. For action anticipation, the results have improved slightly for DINOv2 and VideoMAE, compared to our validation set. It is also notable that the results for the two tasks are roughly at the same level, and for DINOv2, the results for anticipation are even slightly better than those for the recognition task. Surprisingly, ActionCLIP yields the worst performance on this test set, although it produced the best and most balanced combined accuracy scores in Table 1 using the validation set.

Table 2. Results of the three foundation models on the official test set for the T3 Challenge 2025. Top-1 accuracies are reported separately for recognition, anticipation, and the combination. Bold font highlights the best overall results.

	Recognition	Anticipation	Total
Model	Top-1	Top-1	Top-1
DINOv2	**30.50%**	**30.73%**	**30.61%**
VideoMAE	30.24%	29.11%	29.69%
ActionCLIP	25.03%	24.66%	24.85%

Overall, DINOv2 slightly outperforms VideoMAE in all three metrics, with an overall top-1 accuracy of 30.61%. However, the difference between the two methods is very small at only 0.9% on average. The poor performance of ActionCLIP on the 2025 T3 test set suggests that it could not fully utilize its zero-shot capabilities. Note that we limited the training to a relatively small number of epochs due to time constraints. We expect slightly improved results with longer training schedules.

Investigating the individual results in more detail reveals that all models likely struggle with the same videos. In general, only a few videos are classified with moderate accuracy for both recognition and anticipation. Instead, the performance on all clips of a video tends to be either strong or poor. This could be a result of the test set composition, as it contains two types of videos: 36 unseen regular procedure videos and 43 just-in-time procedure videos. The just-in-time procedure videos, in particular, present a substantial challenge for the models, contributing to the pronounced performance gap between the test and validation sets. The results also suggest that the models learn frequently occurring classes in the training set reasonably well, whereas rare edge cases, particularly classes with only one or two samples, remain poorly modeled.

5 Conclusion

We adapted and evaluated three widely known foundation models – DINOv2, VideoMAE, and ActionCLIP – on the recognition and anticipation of medical procedure actions as part of the T3 Challenge 2025. The models reflect three different methods of processing the video information: frame-based, video-based, and a multi-modal approach based on video and text. We first adapted the three models to the challenge task, investigating prompt handling, hyperparameters, and loss weighting. Our evaluation indicates that the three foundation models show a decent performance on the recognition task and perform strongly with multiple possible predictions (top-5 accuracy). On the official test set, DINOv2 yields the best results with an overall accuracy of 30.61%. Despite this limited overall accuracy on the test set, our evaluation indicates the potential of foundation models in this data-scarce medical application with as few as one or two samples per class.

Disclosure of Interests. The authors have no competing interests to declare that are relevant to the content of this article.

References

1. Arnab, A., Dehghani, M., Heigold, G., Sun, C., Lučić, M., Schmid, C.: ViViT: a video vision transformer. In: International Conference on Computer Vision (2021)
2. Awais, M., et al.: Foundation models defining a new era in vision: a survey and outlook. IEEE Trans. Pattern Anal. Mach. Intell. (2025)
3. Caron, M., et al.: Emerging properties in self-supervised vision transformers. In: International Conference on Computer Vision (2021)
4. Carreira, J., Zisserman, A.: Quo vadis, action recognition? A new model and the Kinetics Dataset, In: Computer Vision and Pattern Recognition (2017)
5. Cubuk, E.D., Zoph, B., Shlens, J., Le, Q.V.: Randaugment: practical automated data augmentation with a reduced search space. In: Proceedings of the IEEE/CVF Conference on Computer Vision and Pattern Recognition Workshops, pp. 702–703 (2020)

6. Darcet, T., Oquab, M., Mairal, J., Bojanowski, P.: Vision transformers need registers. In: International Conference on Learning Representations (2024)
7. Dollar, P., Rabaud, V., Cottrell, G., Belongie, S.: Behavior recognition via sparse spatio-temporal features. In: International Workshop on Visual Surveillance and Performance Evaluation of Tracking and Surveillance (2005)
8. Donahue, J., et al.: Long-term recurrent convolutional networks for visual recognition and description. IEEE Trans. Pattern Anal. Mach. Intell. **39**(4), 677–691 (2017)
9. Dosovitskiy, A., et al.: An image is worth 16x16 words: transformers for image recognition at scale. In: International Conference on Learning Representations (2021)
10. Feichtenhofer, C., Pinz, A., Zisserman, A.: Convolutional two-stream network fusion for video action recognition. In: Computer Vision and Pattern Recognition (2016)
11. Gerhardt, R.T., Berry, J.A., Blackbourne, L.H.: Analysis of life-saving interventions performed by out-of-hospital combat medical personnel. J. Trauma Acute Care Surg. **71**(1) (2011)
12. He, K., Chen, X., Xie, S., Li, Y., Dollár, P., Girshick, R.: Masked autoencoders are scalable vision learners. In: Computer Vision and Pattern Recognition (2022)
13. Kay, W., et al.: The kinetics human action video dataset. arXiv preprint-arXiv:1705.06950 (2017)
14. Oakden-Rayner, L.: Exploring large-scale public medical image datasets. Acad. Radiol. **27**(1) (2020)
15. Oquab, M., et al.: DINOv2: learning robust visual features without supervision. Trans. Mach. Learn. Res. (2024)
16. Radford, A., et al.: Learning transferable visual models from natural language supervision. In: International Conference on Machine Learning (2021)
17. Tong, Z., Song, Y., Wang, J., Wang, L.: VideoMAE: masked autoencoders are data-efficient learners for self-supervised video pre-training. In: Advances in Neural Information Processing Systems (2022)
18. Tran, D., Bourdev, L., Fergus, R., Torresani, L., Paluri, M.: Learning spatiotemporal features with 3D convolutional networks. In: International Conference on Computer Vision (2015)
19. Wang, L., et al.: Temporal segment networks for action recognition in videos. IEEE Trans. Pattern Anal. Mach. Intell. **41**(11) (2018)
20. Wang, M., Xing, J., Liu, Y.: ActionCLIP: a new paradigm for video action recognition (2021)
21. Yuan, L., et al.: VideoGLUE: video general understanding evaluation of foundation models. Trans. Mach. Learn. Res. (2023)
22. Zhou, J., et al.: iBOT: Image bert pre-training with online tokenizer. In: International Conference on Learning Representations (2022)
23. Zhuo, Y., et al.: The trauma thompson challenge (2025). https://t3challenge25.grand-challenge.org/. Accessed 11 Sept 2025
24. Zhuo, Y., Zhang, E., Yu, X., et al.: An egocentric life-saving interventional procedure dataset of actions, medical questions, maneuvers and tools. Sci. Data **13**, 51 (2026). https://doi.org/10.1038/s41597-025-06365-y

YOLOv10-Based Multi-task Framework for Hand Localization and Laterality Classification in Surgical Videos

Kedi Sun and Le Zhang(✉)

School of Engineering, College of Engineering and Physical Sciences, University of Birmingham, Birmingham, UK
kxs1163@student.bham.ac.uk, l.zhang.16@bham.ac.uk

Abstract. Real-time hand tracking in trauma surgery is essential for supporting rapid and precise intraoperative decisions. We propose a YOLOv10-based framework that simultaneously localizes hands and classifies their laterality (left or right) in complex surgical scenes. The model is trained on the Trauma THOMPSON Challenge 2025 Task 2 dataset, consisting of first-person surgical videos with annotated hand bounding boxes. Extensive data augmentation and a multi-task detection design improve robustness against motion blur, lighting variations, and diverse hand appearances. Evaluation demonstrates accurate left-hand (67%) and right-hand (71%) classification, while distinguishing hands from the background remains challenging. The model achieves an $mAP_{[0.5:0.95]}$ of 0.33 and maintains real-time inference, highlighting its potential for intraoperative deployment. This work establishes a foundation for advanced hand-instrument interaction analysis in emergency surgical procedures.

Keywords: Hand Tracking · YOLOv10 · Real-Time Detection · Surgical Video · Multi-Task Learning · Trauma Surgery

1 Introduction

Hand tracking in medical emergency procedures is an emerging yet critical research problem in computer-assisted intervention. In urgent and high-stakes scenarios, surgeons and care providers must rapidly identify and manipulate appropriate medical tools while maintaining precise hand coordination. The ability to automatically and reliably capture hand movements, classify hand laterality (left or right), and recognize surgical instruments in real time can substantially enhance intraoperative decision-making and reduce the likelihood of adverse events.

At the 28th International Conference on Medical Image Computing and Computer Assisted Intervention (MICCAI) 2025, the Trauma THOMPSON Challenge Task 2 was introduced to advance the field of emergency procedure analysis. This task addresses the critical problem of real-time hand tracking and tool

J. P. Wachs et al. (Eds.): TrackRAD/TTC 2025, LNCS 16474, pp. 126–132, 2027.
https://doi.org/10.1007/978-3-032-35046-6_12

recognition in trauma care [1]. Building upon previous efforts in surgical tool detection and hand-object interaction understanding, this competition extends the scope to include precise hand localization, laterality classification (left versus right hand), and instrument identification under the unpredictable conditions of trauma surgery.

The challenge provides a unique dataset collected from diverse trauma procedure recordings, characterized by multiple hand appearances, rapid hand movements, and complex hand-tool interactions. With the largest curated dataset of its kind in emergency medicine, annotated by clinical experts, the Trauma THOMPSON Challenge 2025 offers a standardized platform for benchmarking and encourages the development of multi-task learning models that can improve robustness and generalizability.

In this work, we adopt YOLOv10 [2] as the core detection backbone due to its balance between detection accuracy and real-time inference speed, which is essential in emergency surgical scenarios. Building upon YOLOv10, we have implemented a series of improvements, such as task-specific class definitions, a multi-task detection paradigm, and data augmentation for robustness. During training and validation, model performance was primarily assessed using mean Average Precision (mAP) at different Intersection-over-Union (IoU) thresholds, following the COCO protocol, with both $mAP_{0.5}$ and $mAP_{[0.5:0.95]}$ reported. In addition, precision, recall, and F1-score were monitored to provide a balanced evaluation of false positives and false negatives. Final model selection was based on the highest $mAP_{[0.5:0.95]}$, with the F1-score serving as an auxiliary measure of robustness.

2 Methods

2.1 Dataset

The Trauma THOMPSON Challenge includes 5 tasks. Among these, the dataset for Task 2 consists of 20 different surgical videos, filmed from the surgeon's first-person perspective [1]. Each video lasts approximately 40 s, with hand bounding boxes annotated in COCO format. During training, we first cleaned the data by removing three videos with poorly annotated hand movements and converted the videos into images frame-by-frame for training using the YOLOv10 framework. We then divided the remaining dataset into an 80% training set (15 videos) and a 20% test set (2 videos).

2.2 Model Architectures

The proposed framework is built upon YOLOv10, a well-developed object detection model known for its favorable trade-off between detection accuracy and inference speed [2]. This property makes it particularly suitable for real-time applications in trauma surgery, where rapid decision-making is essential. The network follows the conventional one-stage detector design, consisting of a backbone for feature extraction, a neck for multi-scale feature aggregation, and a detection head for bounding box regression and class prediction.

To adapt YOLOv10 to the requirements of our task, we extended the output space to explicitly include "left hand" and "right hand" as distinct categories. This modification allows the model to simultaneously localize hands, classify their laterality, and recognize interacting instruments within a unified detection framework. In practice, this design enables multi-task detection without significant overhead, while ensuring consistency with the downstream evaluation metrics of the challenge.

In addition, we employ data augmentation strategies such as random flipping, scaling, rotation, and color jittering to enhance robustness against the diverse visual conditions encountered in surgical environments, including variations in viewpoint, motion blur, and lighting. With these adaptations, the YOLOv10-based architecture provides a solid foundation for accurate and efficient hand tracking in real-world emergency settings [3,4].

2.3 Training and Testing

During training, due to computational limitations, all input images were resized to a fixed resolution of 416 × 416 pixels. Extensive data augmentation was applied, including random flipping, scaling, rotation, and color jittering. This enhances robustness against variations in viewpoint, lighting, and motion blur commonly encountered in trauma surgery. In addition, the model was optimized using stochastic gradient descent (SGD) with an initial learning rate of 0.01, momentum of 0.9, and weight decay of 0.05.

A cosine annealing scheduler was employed to progressively decrease the learning rate over time [5]. The training process was conducted in 2 rounds, each for 30 epochs with a batch size of 8. To mitigate overfitting, several strategies were adopted: a dropout layer with a rate of 0.2 was introduced to regularize feature learning [6], an early stopping criterion with patience 10 was applied to terminate training when validation performance plateaued, and mosaic augmentation was disabled during the final 10 epochs to improve convergence stability. Model checkpoints were saved periodically, and the best-performing checkpoint was selected based on the highest $mAP_{[0.5:0.95]}$ score on the validation set.

For testing, the trained model was applied to unseen sequences without any test-time augmentation to evaluate its generalization capability under realistic conditions. Performance was assessed using mAP, precision, recall, and F1-score, in accordance with the official challenge protocol [7]. In addition, inference speed was measured in frames per second (FPS), ensuring that the model met the real-time requirements necessary for deployment in trauma surgery assistance systems.

2.4 Ablation Studies and Comparative Analysis

To better understand the contribution of different components in our proposed framework, we conducted ablation studies focusing on three key aspects: (i) hand laterality classification, (ii) data augmentation strategies, and (iii) regularization methods.

1. **Laterality classification:** When the model was trained without distinguishing left and right hands, the overall detection $mAP_{[0.5:0.95]}$ slightly improved to 0.36, suggesting that laterality prediction introduces additional complexity. However, this simplified design sacrifices clinically relevant information, as distinguishing left from right hands is critical in surgical workflows. Thus, our final model retained explicit laterality classification despite the minor performance trade-off.
2. **Data augmentation:** We compared models trained with and without augmentation. Without augmentation, the $mAP_{[0.5:0.95]}$ dropped to 0.27, and recall decreased to below 0.50, highlighting the necessity of augmentation in handling motion blur, occlusion, and lighting variations common in trauma surgery. Notably, random flipping and scaling contributed most significantly to robustness, whereas color jittering had only marginal benefits.
3. **Regularization strategies:** The use of dropout ($p = 0.2$) and early stopping improved validation stability, reducing overfitting compared to baseline training. In contrast, when dropout was removed, validation loss increased sharply after 20 epochs, and final $mAP_{[0.5:0.95]}$ dropped by ~ 0.04. This confirms the importance of regularization in maintaining generalizability under limited training data conditions.

Beyond ablations, we compared YOLOv10 with two alternative detection backbones: YOLOv8 and DETR. YOLOv8 achieved a slightly higher $mAP_{[0.5:0.95]}$ of 0.35 but suffered from slower inference speed (~ 28 FPS versus YOLOv10's ~ 38 FPS), making it less suitable for real-time deployment. DETR achieved competitive accuracy on static frames but failed to meet the real-time requirement (< 10 FPS). These comparisons emphasize that YOLOv10 strikes a favorable balance between accuracy and speed, which is essential in emergency care scenarios where latency can directly impact patient outcomes.

3 Results

The training and validation performance of the proposed YOLOv10-based framework are illustrated in Fig. 1. During training, the box loss, classification loss, and distribution focal loss decreased steadily, indicating that the network successfully learned meaningful feature representations [2]. However, the validation losses exhibited a gradual increase after the early epochs, suggesting the presence of mild overfitting despite the regularization strategies adopted.

In terms of detection performance, the model achieved a stable $mAP_{[0.5:0.95]}$ of approximately 0.33 on the validation set. The $mAP_{0.5}$ reached values above 0.65, demonstrating that the detector was effective in localizing hands under relaxed IoU thresholds. Precision and recall fluctuated during training, stabilizing around 0.58–0.60 recall and 0.80–0.85 precision, which indicates that the model maintains a reasonable balance between false positives and false negatives [7].

Figure 2 shows the probability of correct recognition for the left hand and right hand. The normalized confusion matrix indicates that the model achieves

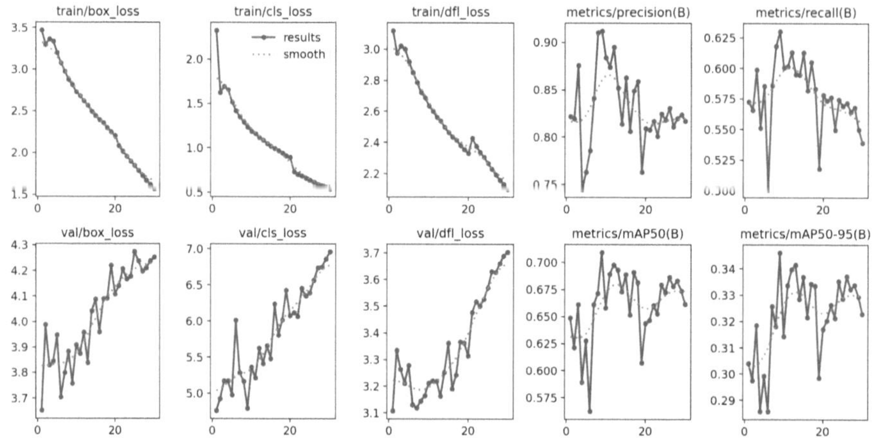

Fig. 1. Curves of various assessment indicators in the final round of training.

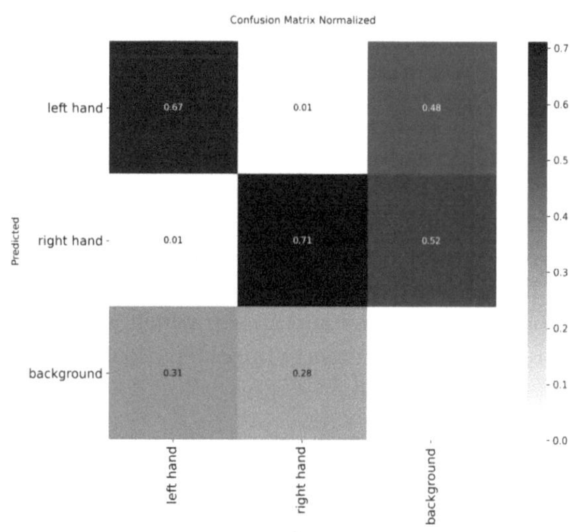

Fig. 2. The normalized confusion matrix of the final training round.

reasonable performance in classifying hand laterality, with 67% of left-hand and 71% of right-hand instances correctly recognized [8]. Misclassifications mainly occur between hand laterality and the background, with left-hand actions being confused with the background 31% of the time, and right-hand actions 28% of the time. The background class is also prone to being misclassified as left or right hand actions [9]. Overall, while the model effectively distinguishes between left and right hand movements, its ability to separate hand actions from background remains limited, suggesting that further refinement or additional background features may improve classification performance.

4 Discussion and Conclusion

In this work, we presented a YOLOv10-based framework for real-time hand tracking in trauma surgery, with explicit classification of left and right hands. The results demonstrate that the model achieves reasonable detection and classification performance, particularly in distinguishing hand laterality [10], with 67% of left-hand and 71% of right-hand actions correctly recognized.

Figure 3 and Fig. 4 show the actual results. However, the confusion matrix indicates persistent misclassification between hand actions and background regions, suggesting that hand-background separation remains a key challenge in complex surgical scenes.

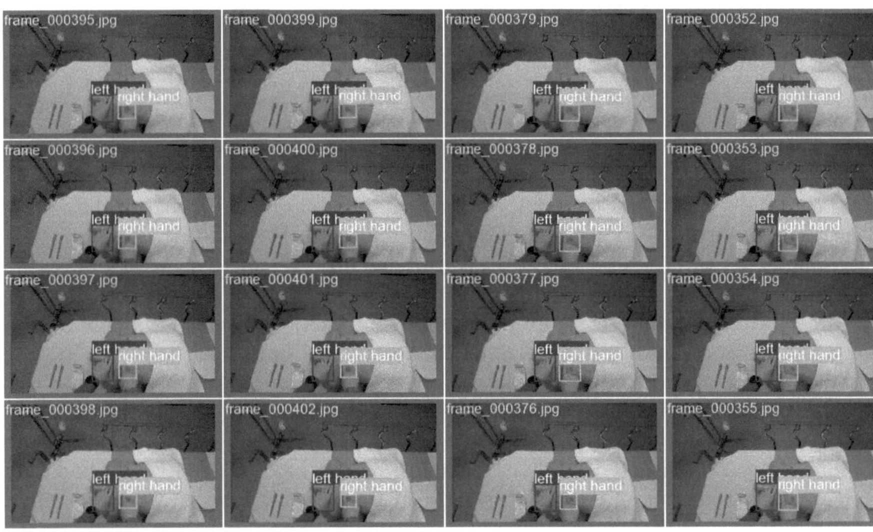

Fig. 3. Model performance on the test set.

The $mAP_{[0.5:0.95]}$ of approximately 0.33 highlights that, while the model can localize hands effectively under relaxed IoU thresholds ($mAP_{0.5} > 0.65$), tighter

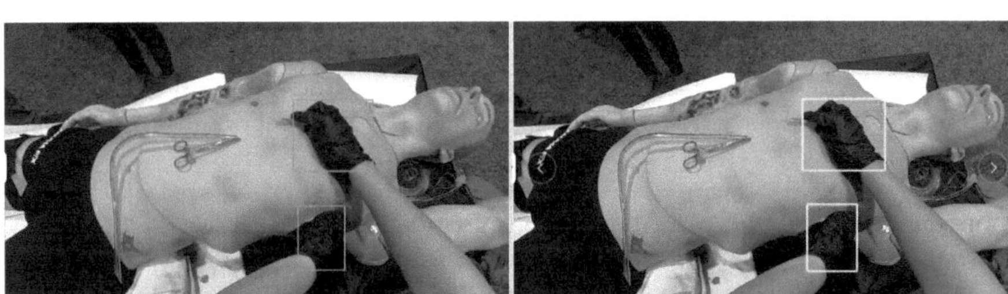

Fig. 4. Comparison of actual model performance (left) and Ground Truth (right).

localization requirements still expose limitations in precision. Precision and recall values (0.80–0.85 and 0.58–0.60, respectively) further indicate that the model favors reducing false positives over false negatives, which may be acceptable in safety-critical medical scenarios where detecting all hand movements is prioritized. The overfitting observed in the validation losses suggests that future work could benefit from larger, more diverse datasets, improved regularization strategies, or temporal information integration to enhance robustness.

Overall, the proposed framework demonstrates the feasibility of leveraging real-time object detection models for multi-task hand tracking in trauma care. The approach can serve as a foundation for subsequent improvements, including integrating temporal modeling [11], enhancing background discrimination [10], or extending the framework to simultaneous hand-instrument interaction analysis [12]. Such advancements could further support intraoperative decision-making, reduce cognitive load on surgeons, and contribute to safer, more efficient trauma procedures.

References

1. Zhuo, Y., et al.: An Egocentric life-saving interventional procedure dataset of actions, medical questions. Maneuvers and tools. Sci. Data (2025)
2. Wang, A., et al.: Yolov10: Real-time end-to-end object detection. Adv. Neural. Inf. Process. Syst. **37**, 107984–108011 (2024)
3. Ulmer, M.: How important are data augmentations to close the domain gap for object detection in orbit? In: 2025 IEEE Aerospace Conference. IEEE (2025)
4. Zhao, L., et al.: Maximum-entropy adversarial data augmentation for improved generalization and robustness. Adv. Neural. Inf. Process. Syst. **33**, 14435–14447 (2020)
5. Johny, A., Madhusoodanan, K.: Dynamic learning rate in deep CNN model for metastasis detection and classification of histopathology images. Comput. Math. Methods Med. **2021**(1), 5557168 (2021)
6. Srivastava, N., et al.: Dropout: a simple way to prevent neural networks from overfitting. J. Mach. Learn. Res. **15**(1), 1929–1958 (2014)
7. Davis, J., Goadrich, M.: The relationship between Precision-Recall and ROC curves. In: Proceedings of the 23rd International Conference on Machine Learning (2006)
8. Wang, J., et al.: Rgb2hands: real-time tracking of 3d hand interactions from monocular RGB video. ACM Trans. Graph. (ToG) **39**(6), 1–16 (2020)
9. Zhang, F.: Mediapipe hands: on-device real-time hand tracking. arXiv preprint arXiv:2006.10214 (2020)
10. Fujii, R., Saito, H., Kajita, H.: EgoSurgery-tool: a dataset of surgical tool and hand detection from egocentric open surgery videos. arXiv preprintarXiv:2406.03095 (2024)
11. Simonyan, K., Zisserman, A.: Two-stream convolutional networks for action recognition in videos. Adv. Neural. Inf. Process. Syst. **27** (2014)
12. Twinanda, A.P., et al.: Endonet: a deep architecture for recognition tasks on laparoscopic videos. IEEE Trans. Med. Imaging **36**(1), 86–97 (2016)

Author Index

J. P. Wachs et al. (Eds.): TrackRAD/TTC 2025, LNCS 16474, p. 133, 2027.
https://doi.org/10.1007/978-3-032-35046-6

MIX
Papier aus verantwortungsvollen Quellen
Paper from responsible sources
FSC® C105338
FSC
www.fsc.org

If you have any concerns about our products,
you can contact us on
ProductSafety@springernature.com

In case Publisher is established outside the EU,
the EU authorized representative is:
Springer Nature Customer Service Center GmbH
Europaplatz 3, 69115 Heidelberg, Germany

Printed by Libri Plureos GmbH
in Hamburg, Germany